TOMLINSON, Max

Clean up your diet

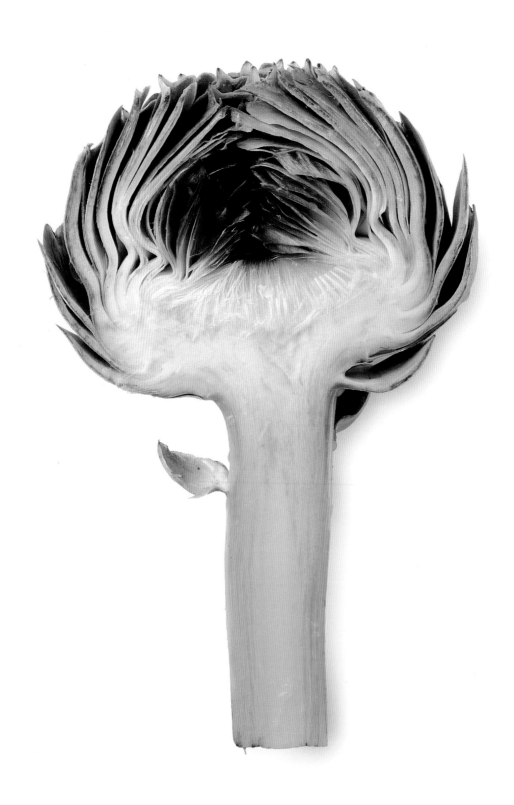

CLEAN UP YUR DIET

The pure food
programme to cleanse,
energize and revitalize

MAX TOMLINSON

dbp

DUNCAN BAIRD PUBLISHERS

LONDON

Clean Up Your Diet
MAX TOMLINSON

First published in the United Kingdom
and Ireland in 2007 by
Duncan Baird Publishers Ltd
Sixth Floor
Castle House
75–76 Wells Street
London W1T 3QH

Conceived, created and designed by
Duncan Baird Publishers Ltd

Recipes created with Caroline Brewester.

Managing Designer: Manisha Patel
Designer: Luana Gobbo
Managing Editor: Grace Cheetham
Editor: Judy Barratt
Recipe editor: Gillian Haslam
Commissioned Photography: Simon Smith and
Toby Scott
Photographic assistants: Michael Hart, Matthew McCully and
Tom Alexander

British Library Cataloguing-in-Publication Data:
A CIP record for this book is available from the
British Library.

ISBN: 978-1-84483-362-7

10 9 8 7 6 5 4 3 2

Typeset in Frutiger and Transitional
Colour reproduction by Scanhouse, Malaysia
Printed in Thailand by Imago

Publisher's note

Before following any advice or practice suggested in this
book, it is recommended that you consult a medical
practitioner as to its suitability, especially if you suffer from
any health problems or special conditions, or if you are
pregnant. The publishers, author and photographers cannot
accept any responsibility for any injuries or damage incurred
as a result of using any of the therapeutic methods described
or mentioned here.

Recipe measurements – Australia

The recipe ingredients in this book are given in metric,
imperial, and US cup measurements. Please note that where
tablespoons are used, an Australian tablespoon is 25% larger
than a US/UK tablespoon. If you are in Australia you should
adjust the quantity downward by 25% (2 tbsp becomes
1½ tbsp and so on).

Dedication

To Filipa, Jaspar and Ava – life means a whole lot more since you arrived in mine.

To my family: Mom, Cam and Dad – thanks for believing and caring.

To my friends, extended family and colleagues – love and respect.

To Grace, Borra, Judy and Caroline – the best team ever.

To Cisca – for starting me off.

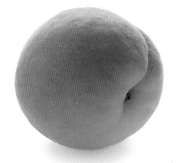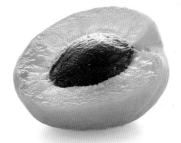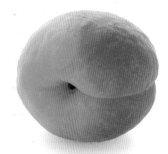

CONTENTS

KEY

The following symbols are used to indicate the
nutritional content of the recipes in this book.

Ⓥ	vegetarian	Ⓞ	contains eggs
Ⓧ	gluten-free	Ⓟ	high in iron
Ⓧ	wheat-free	Ⓞ	high in omega-3s
Ⓓ	dairy-free	Ⓒ	high in calcium

FOREWORD

I remember very clearly the first time I realized that I wanted to be a naturopath. I was 12 years old and had just bought *The Nature Doctor* by the renowned Swiss naturopathic doctor Alfred Vogel. As I read I was astounded by the depth of my feelings and the way his ideas and words seemed to make perfect sense, as if I already knew what naturopathy (or "nature cure" as he put it) was. I sat on the verandah of our house in Cape Town, dreaming of the day I could meet Dr Vogel and start to explore the world of natural medicine. Years later I did visit Switzerland, but he was very old and frail by this time and I was not able to meet him. I suppose in some way this book is my tribute to the original naturopathic masters – the men and women who opened all of our eyes to the power that nature has to heal. Lindlahr, Jensen, Vogel, Kneipp, Shelton, Bircher-Benner – all great healers. Thank you.

Sydney, Australia, was where I finally qualified as a naturopath. I stepped out with a whole arsenal of vitamins, minerals, herbs and homoeopathics at my disposal and I travelled the world meeting natural healers and doctors, expanding my knowledge of herbs and modern orthomolecular nutrition, priding myself on my ability to apply science to my natural therapies' practice. Something was missing, though, and the results I was getting with clients reflected this. I was a very modern naturopath – but I had forgotten about a diet of plain, simple food as the basis of all health.

After several more years' research, I realized that food was the key to lasting wellbeing. I learned how tomatoes and cabbage can fight against cancer, garlic can lower blood pressure, apple-skin and onions can reduce the risk of heart attack – and much, much more besides. It was soon clear to me that food has an amazing power to heal – but also that not all food contains the nutrients and natural chemicals we need. The way that we grow produce, transport, process, store and cook our food all have an impact on the quality of our diet.

This book is the result of my research for the perfect, pure foods that contain all of the nutrients we need to maintain health in the human body. I have come to the conclusion that the way to clean up our diets is to fill them with organic, seasonal and properly cooked foods that burst with nutritional value.

In this book I show you how to use simple dietary principles to detox your body, correct the functioning of your digestive tract, and re-energize your day. In addition, I show you how to maintain all the good nutritional work you are doing for yourself well into the future to keep you happier, healthier, younger-looking and younger-feeling to the end of your days. My journey started 28 years ago; your journey to optimum health starts now. I sincerely hope you enjoy it as much as I did.

Max Tomlinson
August 2006

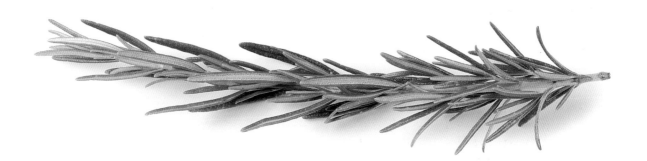

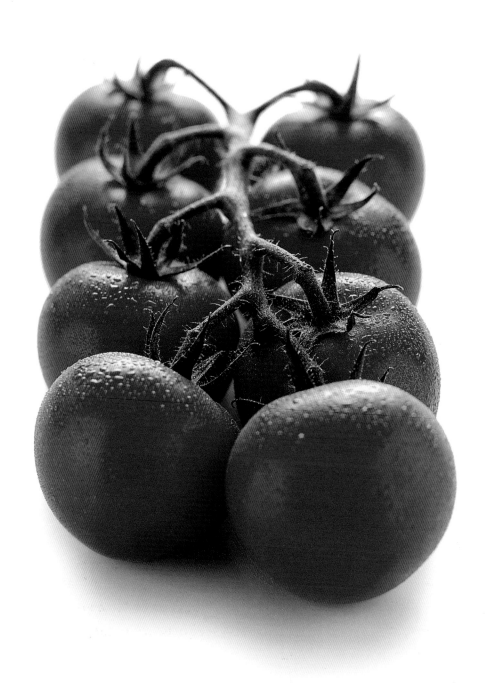

CHAPTER 1

Principles of a clean diet

Your health – physical, mental and emotional – depends largely on what you put into your body. For most of us with busy lives and pressing schedules, what we put in are convenience foods, which require the least amount of preparation and cooking. However, apart from being quick to put together, these foods really have little to recommend them; they offer a reduced number of nutrients – the vitamins and minerals that we need to be healthy – and an abundance of additives, the combination of which may damage our health. This chapter will provide you with the basic knowledge you need to clean up your diet. It will show you how many of the foods available today have, through modern farming practices, as well as processing and packaging, become nutrient-depleted. Then it will show you how a return to pure, natural foods, grown, cooked and presented as nature intended, can bring us back to a state of optimum health, so that we look and feel great well into our future.

WHAT IS A CLEAN DIET?

How would you like to wake up every morning raring to go? When did you last burst with energy all day long? Wouldn't it be great if your clothes didn't feel tight and uncomfortable after a meal? A clean diet rich with pure foods makes all this possible.

Food through time

We have to go back only a hundred years or so to see how different were the diets of our ancestors from our own diets today. Before massive urbanization led to a move away from farm-fresh, natural foods and toward modern, processed foods, our ancestors generally ate from the land and the immediate surroundings, benefiting from fresh and mostly organic produce. Farmers and gardeners returned essential nutrients to the land by mulching, adding manure, and crop rotation, all of which served to maintain the quality of the soil, and in turn the quality of the plants that grew in it and the animals that fed on it.

All this began to change after World War II, when companies that had once made weapons instead used their chemicals in fertilizers. They promised farmers a way to maximize the growth of crops and animals, and to minimize the nuisance of insects. Today, US farmers use around 1.4 billion kg (3 billion lb) of pesticides on their crops. These farm chemicals end up in the food chain, with some authorities estimating that up to 45 per cent of vegetables on sale contain traces of pesticides. To make matters worse, chemical fertilizers strip the soil of its essential nutrients, including calcium (which we need for healthy bones), magnesium (for energy, and muscle function), and selenium (for our heart). If these nutrients are not present in the soil, they cannot be present in the foods that grow in them. Some sources say that mineral levels in our commercial foods have fallen by more than 40 per cent in the last 50 years.

Finally in this unhappy tale of modern food, we have to look at transportation and food-processing. The longer it takes for food to reach our table, the fewer essential nutrients there will be in it. In particular vitamins A and C degrade over time. Food-processing strips away other nutrients. Processing meat reduces the levels of vitamin B6 (essential for immunity and brain function) by up to 70 per cent. Freezing meat can destroy up to 50 per cent of the vitamin-B1 and -B2 content (both important energy nutrients).

Cleaning up with "pure" foods

Naturopaths have always said that you are what you eat – it may be a cliché, but it's true. Cleaning up your diet means thinking about what you put into your body, and its effects on you. That goes for the kinds of food you eat (the quarter-pounder versus a lean breast of chicken), but also – and more importantly – the quality of the foods you eat. I'm not talking about just the standard, "healthier" options in terms of food type, but foods that are better in terms of their nutrients. Indeed, I would rather you ate a homemade quarter-pounder, containing 100-per-cent organic, lean minced beef, fresh, organic herbs, and immune-boosting organic onion (with a free-range, organic egg to bind them together) than a chicken breast from a battery-farmed, non-organic hen, which is likely to be severely nutrient-depleted.

The answer to cleaning up your diet lies in simple, "pure foods" – and you will see that phrase pop up in this book time and again. These foods are the healthiest options in terms of the kinds of food that you choose to eat, but they are also grown, farmed or cultivated using the most nutrient-rich methods – organically, with the minimum amount of transport time and processing.

Why are pure foods better for us?

Over the course of the plans (chapters 2, 3 and 4) in this book, the benefits of cleaning up your diet will become increasingly clear. For now, though, let's look at the main reasons why pure foods are the best option.

HEALTHY BODY SYSTEMS Although it sounds obvious, providing more of the nutrients your body needs to function optimally is the fastest route to improved health and wellbeing. Pure foods are free from the additives and chemicals that in modern processed foods place such a strain on the organs of elimination, such as the liver and kidneys. They are also rich in essential micronutrients (vitamins and minerals, plant nutrients called phytonutrients, and other beneficial organisms, such as probiotics, or healthy bacteria), which they provide in a form that the body finds easy to absorb. This helps to ease the work of the digestive system, making it more efficient at getting all the goodness into your blood stream and so around your body. Finally, pure foods are well-balanced in terms of their carbohydrate content, which means that they act to stabilize energy levels throughout the day.

FIGHTING ILLNESS The blood carries nutrients to the main parts of your immune system, including the lymph nodes (glands), spleen and thymus gland, which work together to produce special cells called lymphocytes. The lymphocytes attack antigens – invading bacteria, viruses or fungi that can cause illness. As well as providing the most nutrients (particularly vitamins A and C) for the immune system, pure foods provide the fewest toxins (pesticides, preservatives and so on) that compromise immune function. Pure foods are also rich in antioxidants – natural plant chemicals that help to neutralize free radicals, which can cause cancer (see p.36). Finally, a diet rich in a diverse range of pure foods helps to reduce the risk of developing a food sensitivity, which is often purely the result of overexposure to the same, nutrient-depleted foods, which causes an oversensitive reaction in your immune system. As well as their general immune-boosting effects, we can use pure foods to optimize specific nutrients in our diet to fight specific conditions – for example, increasing our intake of calcium to fight osteoarthritis (see p.185) or magnesium to reduce the effects of asthma (see p.166). Pure foods are pure medicine.

KEEPING SLIM AND YOUNG Finally, pure foods help to keep us in peak condition. They provide a balanced diet, free from sugar and saturated fat, which helps your weight to stabilize. They also provide lots of antioxidants, which reduce the risk of developing cancer, and also help to prevent free radicals from damaging cells in the skin, hair and nails – the cause of the visible signs of ageing. By optimizing the function of all our body systems, pure foods prolong their efficiency and reduce the likelihood of developing age-related illnesses, such as heart disease, brittle bones, and dementia.

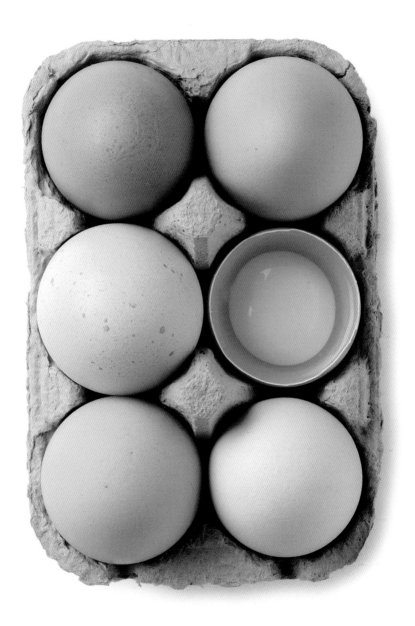

SEVEN STEPS TO A CLEAN DIET

Now that you have a sense of what it means to clean up your diet – by eating pure foods rich with nutrients – and so optimize your health, it's time to get down to the nitty gritty. What follows are the seven steps you'll need to take when you buy or cook your food to ensure that you are eating the clean, "pure foods" way.

1 Go organic

Commercial farming methods use an array of chemicals to protect crops and promote growth in plants and animals. Some of these manmade chemicals are now thought to cause disease (including some cancers), as well as hyperactivity in children, and asthma, eczema and a host of other illnesses; others upset our hormonal balance, leading to problems such as infertility or mood swings. Organic farmers avoid using toxic chemical sprays on their crops, and their animals are kept in more natural, free-range conditions and are fed on natural foods. In addition organic meat does not come from animals that have been "beefed up" using chemical hormones or antibiotics.

Organic foods are strictly regulated by government agencies. As a result you can be sure that when you buy organic you are buying food that has:

• No nasty chemical additives
• No pesticides or insecticides
• No genetically modified (GM) ingredients or additives
• Higher nutrient levels, including vitamin C, and minerals such as calcium
• Far fewer pharmaceutical drugs pumped into it during animal husbandry

(organic farmers use drugs on their animals only when they are sick; whereas conventional farmers may use drugs to promote animals' growth)
• Less of an impact on wildlife and the environment

SHOPPING FOR ORGANIC FOOD

Consumer demand for high-quality organic food has grown hugely over the last decade. In January 2005 farmers managed 686,100 ha (1.7 million acres) of land to organic standards across the UK. According to the US organic standards agency, the number of organic farmers in the US is increasing at a rate of about 12 per cent a year. This is wonderful news for us and for the environment, because it means that healthier food is reaching more of our tables, that the air we breathe is that bit cleaner and fresher, and that birds, butterflies and their fellow creatures have a safer place to live.

However, there are still plenty of us who need convincing about going organic. The most common reason people give for not buying organic foods is that to do so is too expensive.

I am pleased to say that, as more of us demand organic produce, things are changing, but in the meantime it's merely a matter of prioritizing your body and saving money in other places. Avoid impulse buys, make a shopping list and stick to it, and don't be caught by "multi-buy" special offers. Reduce your weekly "luxury" items. One week without a new CD or a new item of clothing

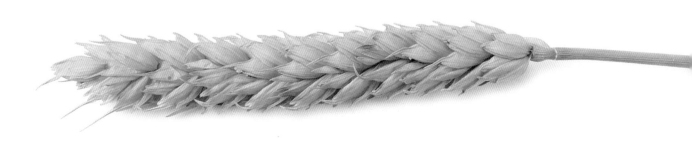

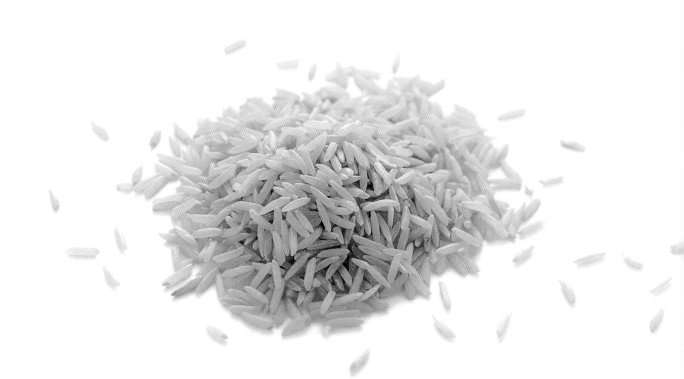

"Pure foods are the nutrient
'spark plugs' that fire up our
health and wellbeing."

will probably pay for a month of going organic. I think you will agree that good food is a great investment!

BOX SCHEMES One great way to get your organic shopping – and to support local producers at the same time – is to sign up to a weekly organic fruit-and-veg box scheme and get a delivery directly from the farm.

2 Go seasonal

It is so easy nowadays for most of us to eat whatever we want, whenever we want it. You need soft, fresh, ripe summer berries in mid-winter? No problem – your local supermarket will have them in stock. The concept of eating what is in season disappeared with the advent of modern food supply and transport, but eating with the seasons is a fundamental naturopathic philosophy and is important because the body needs and craves certain foods depending on the time of year. Winter foods need to be rich and warming, with soups made from organic beans, ginger, herbs, garlic and root vegetables. Summer foods need to be lighter, reflecting the warmth of the time of year. My summertime favourites are massive rainbow-coloured salads and light stir-fries with grilled, organic fish. On the whole, seasonal foods have travelled shorter distances to reach your table and so have suffered less nutrient loss than those that are out of season. You will also find your foods at their tastiest as well as at their most affordable.

FARMERS' MARKETS Take a look in your local newspaper to find a weekly farmers' market in your area. Visit it as part of your weekly shop and choose from the great array of seasonal, fresh foods on sale. Not all the produce at your local market will be organic, of course, but at least you can buy what is truly in season and can also ask the grower directly whether or not he or she overdoes the chemicals on the non-organic produce.

3 Make it fresh

There is no question: fresh is best. Some important vitamins (including vitamins A and C) degrade over time as a result of exposure to light, heat and oxygen. A report conducted by the American Dietetic Association recommends that we should consume orange juice as soon as possible after we buy it, because the vitamin-C content decreases more and more rapidly the closer the product gets to its expiry date. In two weeks the level of vitamin C in one carton generally fell from 65 milligrams per serving to 45 milligrams. The level fell again to about 36 milligrams after four weeks – a reduction of close to 50 per cent. So, when you have a cold or the flu, drinking commercial orange juice to pack your body with vitamin C might not be the best option. However, freshly squeezed orange juice, made from ripe, organic oranges, will supply all the vitamin C you need to fight off the bugs. Apply this attitude on freshness to all your fruit and vegetables and your nutrient intake will soar!

4 Aim for minimally processed, and lightly cooked or raw

Most commercial food-processing methods involve using heat to cook the food and to destroy any resident bacteria, thus prolonging shelf-life. This process destroys or damages some important vitamins and other nutrients that are very sensitive to heat. For example, oil can oxidize (become rancid) when exposed to heat, altering its flavour and smell, and diminishing its nutritional value. More importantly, oxidation produces free radicals (see p.36), which scientists believe play a role in ageing, as well as the development of cancer and other degenerative diseases. Food-processing in the home can also damage nutrients. Correct cooking methods, such as lightly steaming, rather than boiling, or eating foods raw, minimize this damage.

Some vitamins are more stable (less affected by processing, storage and cooking) than others. The water-soluble vitamins (the B-group and C) are more unstable than the fat-soluble vitamins (A, D, E and K) during food-processing and storage. The most unstable vitamins are:

- B1 (thiamine), which is important for mental and emotional wellbeing and to promote good digestion;
- B9 (folic acid), which is important during pregnancy for the healthy growth of the fetus, and for heart and bone health in all of us;
- Vitamin C, which is important as a major stress-buster and immune-booster.

The higher the temperature at which you cook your food, and the longer you cook it, the greater the nutrient loss. According to some sources, cooking to the point of browning or charring creates compounds that are carcinogenic (may cause cancer). Charring proteins (meat, chicken and fish) creates a potentially harmful chemical called heterocyclic aromatic amine, which has been linked with an increased risk of breast cancer among women. Some also say that, while barbecues are great fun, fat dripping into an open flame forms particularly harmful carcinogens called polycyclic aromatic hydrocarbons (PAHs). Cooking food can be a dangerous job! This all sounds very gloomy, but remember that all you need to do to minimize the risks is to eat more raw or lightly cooked produce, and reduce your exposure to charred vegetables and meats. Always cook meat such as chicken all the way through, but don't overcook it. What follows is my guide to cooking pure foods in the right way.

COOKING METHODS – THE NOT SO GOOD

- Boiling. This is my least favourite method of cooking. Boiling toughens the protein in eggs, softens the plant fibre cellulose in cereals, vegetables and fruits, and destroys nutrients. The biggest loss is of minerals into the water. The only vegetable that requires boiling is the potato – steam everything else.

- Deep-frying. Deep-frying involves fully immersing food in hot oil. The main problem with it is the type of oil we use to deep-fry: cooking oil. This is made by treating oils pressed from seeds with chemicals that refine, bleach and then deodorize the oil. This process removes the small percentage of natural plant chemicals that have all of the major health benefits. In addition, the oil degenerates at high temperatures, oxidizing and creating cancer-causing free radicals (see p.36). This is why if you have to deep-fry, you should always use fresh oil, which has not already oxidized. (If you are shallow-frying, use olive oil, which burns at much higher temperatures and so is safer for longer.)

COOKING METHODS – THE GOOD

- Steaming. Light steaming is the best way to cook vegetables and fish. Food is put into a steamer, and, as the water in the lower container boils, steam rises and cooks the food in the upper, perforated pan. Steaming is preferable to boiling as the food loses no minerals at all, and the process does less damage to the food's fragile vitamins and enzymes.

• Dry-frying. This involves cooking without oil in a well-heated, non-stick frying pan (skillet). Add a little water and then add your meat, fish, chicken or vegetables. After a short while, meat and poultry will release their own juices, providing plenty of moisture to prevent burning; as will vegetables. Do not use metal utensils as this damages the non-stick surface in the pan and you end up eating the coating! Try not to overcook your vegetables. They should be crisp and colourful so that they retain their natural flavour and nutrients.

• Stir-frying. Stir-frying involves frying food very quickly over a very high heat in a lightly oiled pan (skillet). It is important to use a good-quality olive oil and not to let the oil burn. Burned oil contains chemicals called free radicals (yes, those again!), which are bad for your health (see p.36). Add a little water as you stir-fry as this helps to spread the oil.

• Oven roasting. The secret to healthy roast vegetables, fish, chicken and meats is not to burn or char them, as this may produce carcinogenic compounds (see p.21). Bear in mind that the longer you cook food for the more nutrients are lost, so it pays to steam your food a little first, partially cooking it quickly, and then to finish it off in the oven.

• Grilling (broiling). This is a great way to prepare fish and lean meats. Pay attention to cooking times and do not burn or char the food. Allow meats to drain as they grill (broil) as this gets rid of excess saturated, unhealthy fats.

• Raw. I am not in favour of a totally raw diet (apologies and respect to anyone who is a raw-fooder), but most of us certainly need to increase the amount of raw food that we eat so that it constitutes about half of our daily intake. Raw, organic salads, fruit and vegetables contain an abundance of vitamins, enzymes (the catalysts for the hundreds of biochemical reactions that occur in the body) and phytochemicals (natural plant nutrients that have a powerful protective action on the body).

FINALLY, CHOOSE YOUR UTENSILS AND CONTAINERS CAREFULLY

The aluminium (aluminum) in cookware leaches into food, accumulating in the brain and nervous system. High brain aluminium levels have been linked to Alzheimer's disease. Foods cooked or stored in aluminium produce a substance

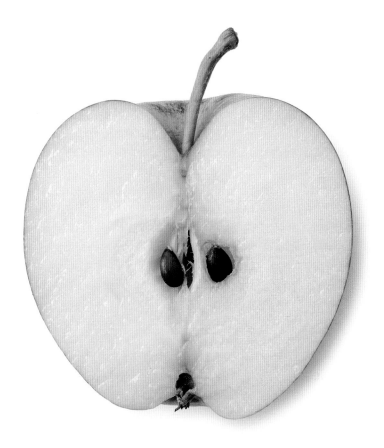

"We lose about 25 per cent of
the vitamin C in vegetables
through boiling food – even for
only a few minutes!"

that neutralizes enzymes in the digestive tract. This can lead to bloating, indigestion, irritable bowel and gastric ulcers. Use stainless steel pans for cooking and plastic tubs for storage (but never leave these in direct sunlight, as if the plastic warms up, it may then leach chemicals into the food).

5 Make food additive-free

More than 12,000 manmade chemicals are added to our foods. In isolation, on rare occasions and in tiny quantities, I'm sure that most of them are fairly benign. What does worry me, though, is that food manufacturers and processors combine any number of chemicals to colour, flavour, enhance and preserve our food. There has been no conclusive research on the effects on our health of the combination of these chemicals – the so-called "cocktail effect" – and when there has been research it tends to have been by the food or additive manufacturers themselves, rather than by independent bodies. From a commonsense, "chemistry" point of view, chemicals act in synergy – react with each other – and create by-products, some of which could be potentially harmful. But how can we know for sure?

Well, unfortunately, we can't – but there's a simple rule for playing safe with additives: read the food labels and don't eat what you can't pronounce. Of course, listing additives by "E numbers", rather than by their names, makes the decisions on what is OK and what is not even more difficult. The list of E numbers given in the box opposite is not complete in any way, and its list of potential side-effects would be long (too long to give here), but it does provide a good basis for identifying the E numbers that you should try to avoid, especially if you are feeding children, whose delicate immune systems tend to be more sensitive to some of these chemicals than those of most adults. However, to give you an idea of what some E numbers can do to you, take a look at these two:

• E239 hexamethylene tetramine. This preservative is a fungicide found in some cheeses and in herring and mackerel. In animal experiments it has been shown to be mutagenic (it causes genetic mutation) and carcinogenic (cancer-causing) and changes to formaldehyde (a type of acid) in the gut. It may cause cancer and kidney disease, and it reduces fertility.

E IS FOR ...

The following table separates the bad from the good in terms of E numbers. The "baddies" are chemical, manmade additives, so are toxic in some way, and I think you should eliminate them from your diet. The "natural alternatives" are additives that come from natural sources and are those additives that I consider "safe". I've given you the names of these, too, so that you can see that many of them are things you will have heard of, or at least that don't sound terrifying or unpronounceable.

THE BADDIES

COLOURS

- E102, E104, E110, E122–E131, E132, E133, E142, E150 (a, b, c, d), E151, E153, E154, E155, E160b

PRESERVATIVES

- E200–E203, E210–E213, E214–E219, E220–E232, E234–E252, E281–E285

ANTIOXIDANTS AND ACIDITY REGULATORS

- E310–E321, E385

THICKENERS, EMULSIFIERS AND STABILIZERS

- E400–E405, E407, E415–E445, E461–E495, E1103

SWEETENERS

- E950–E966

FLAVOUR ENHANCERS

- E621, E627, E631

ANTI-CAKING AGENTS

- E535–E538, E553b

GLAZING AGENTS

- E902, E903, E905c, E914, E915

IMPROVERS AND BLEACHING AGENTS

- E925–E926

OTHERS

- E513, E524–E528

THE NATURAL ALTERNATIVES

COLOURS

- E100 Curcumin, turmeric
- E101 Riboflavin (Vitamin B2)
- E140 Chlorophylls and Chlorophyllins: (i) Chlorophylls (ii) Chlorophyllins
- E160a Beta-carotene
- E160d Lycopene
- E161b Lutein
- E163 Anthocyanins

PRESERVATIVES

- E1105 Lysozyme

ANTIOXIDANTS AND ACIDITY REGULATORS

- E300 Ascorbic acid (Vitamin C)
- E301 Sodium ascorbate
- E302 Calcium ascorbate
- E303 Potassium ascorbate
- E322 Lecithin
- E332 Potassium citrates (i)
- E333 Calcium citrates (i)
- E375 Niacin (nicotinic acid), Nicotinamide

THICKENERS, EMULSIFIERS AND STABILIZERS

- E406 Agar

SWEETENERS

- E967 Xylitol

ANTI-CAKING AGENTS

- E558 Bentonite

GLAZING AGENTS

- E901 Beeswax, white and yellow
- E908 Rice bran wax
- E910 L-cysteine
- E913 Lanolin, sheep wool grease

IMPROVERS

- E920 and E921 L-cysteine

OTHERS

- E948 Oxygen

- E320 Butylated hydroxyanisole (BHA). Food manufacturers use this antioxidant as a preservative in margarine, lard, lemon curd, cakes, pastry, mincemeat, gravy powder, horseradish dips, soft drinks, and chewing gum. It causes cancer in animals, and raises the levels of harmful fats in our blood.

OTHER PROBLEMS ON LABELS

- "Low fat" and its friends. Claims such as "low fat", "reduced sodium" and "high fibre" tend to be commercially driven with no real nutritional basis or strict legal definition. "Lite" and "light" also have no legally binding definition, and are used freely by food manufacturers keen to cash in on no-fat, low-sugar dieters the world over. A clean diet, rich with pure foods, does not need to enhance, remove or replace any of the naturally occurring substances in foods. Fibre is plentiful anyway in pure foods; bad fats, excess salt and simple sugars are scarce. The pure-fooder has no reason to diet, because his or her diet is in perfect balance, which should mean that his or her weight is in perfect balance, too.

- Genetically modified (GM). If you spot the word "modified" on a label, don't buy the product. Genetically modifying food is a brand new science, and this makes me nervous: it takes decades for us to be certain of the effects of food modification on the human body. In addition, GM-containing foods are not always labelled as GM. Many animals are given GM animal feed, but their meat doesn't have to carry a GM label. The only way to be certain to avoid GM meat and poultry is to go organic.

6 Eat the whole grain

Wheat, rye, oats, rice and barley are some of the mainstays of the modern diet. In their wholegrain, natural form, these cereals are a fantastic and very nutritious food. However, modern milling techniques, and the huge worldwide demand for refined, white-flour products, has seen a drastic decline in the nutrient levels in our breads (see p.29), pastas and other cereal-based foods. The sugars in refined grains release quickly into the blood stream, contributing to disorders such as diabetes and to weight-gain. Healthy brown rice, wholemeal pasta, wholemeal brown bread and wholemeal flour are all part of the clean, pure-foods diet.

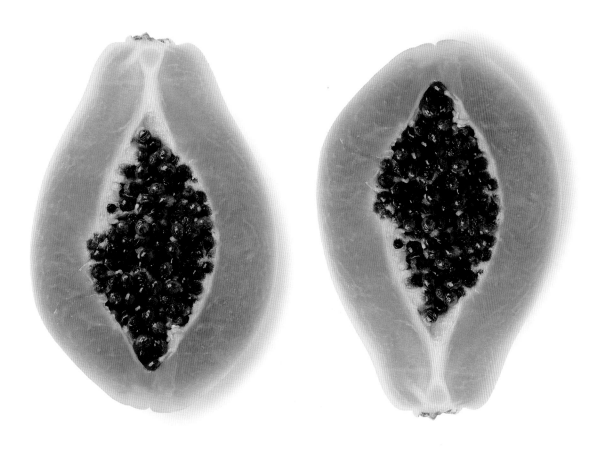

MAX FACT

Over the course of a normal day, the average American consumes more than
180 chemical additives as a result of eating processed food, or unwashed fruit and
vegetables – that's more than 65,000 separate doses of chemical in a year!

PRESERVING THE NUTRIENT VALUE OF FRESH FRUITS AND VEGETABLES

Here are some simple suggestions to help you to retain the maximum nutrient-content in the fruits and vegetables you cook and eat.

• Store foods properly, keeping cold foods cold and sealing oily foods in airtight containers (so that the oils do not come into contact with the air and oxidize).

• Keep vegetables in the crisper section of the refrigerator, which keeps them at just the right temperature to retain their goodness.

• Store fruit away from direct sunlight as sunlight degrades and alters nutrients, especially fragile vitamin A and the good oils.

• Wash and scrub vegetables rather than peeling them (a lot of the nutrients are in or close to the skin). Similarly, wash and use the outer leaves of vegetables like cabbage or lettuce unless they are wilted or unpalatable. Like the skins, the outer leaves contain the highest concentration of some essential nutrients such as vitamin C.

• Steam, roast or grill (broil) vegetables rather than boiling them, and if you do boil your vegetables, save the nutrient-laden water for soup stock.

• Cook foods as quickly as possible as the damage to nutrients increases the longer they spend cooking.

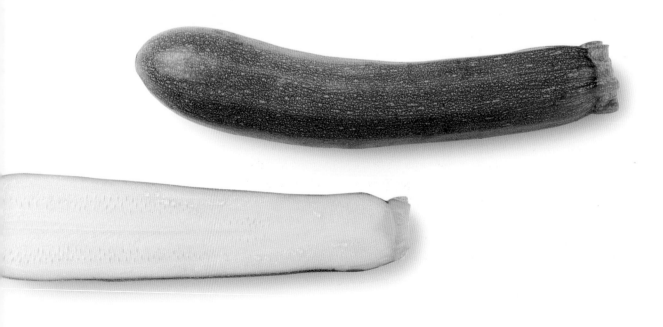

WHOLEGRAIN VS WHITE BREAD

To see just why wholegrain is so important, it pays to take a look at that most humble of foods – bread. Wholegrain wheat is made up of three layers:

- Bran This is the outer, hard coating of the grain of wheat. It is a rich source of dietary fibre (essential for the health of the bowels) and the vitamins B1, B2, B5 and B6 (which help to produce energy and assist with the correct functioning of the nervous system).

- The germ This is a nutrient-, oil-rich kernel containing vitamins E, B1, B2 and B6. (Vitamin E is an important antioxidant, which helps to protect us against cancer and ageing; see p.36.)

- The endosperm This is the bulk of the grain, which supplies protein and carbohydrate. These are essential macronutrients that promote growth and provide fuel for energy, respectively.

Our ancestors ate the "whole" grain, ground up to make fibre- and nutrient-rich wholemeal breads and other wholegrain products. While modern, refined bread does supply carbohydrate and protein (macronutrients), the process of refining removes the outer bran layer and the inner germ, taking with it many of the micronutrients – the fibre, half of the B5, 70 per cent of the B2, most of the B6 and most of the B1.

7 Eat sustainable fish

The clean diet should be healthy for the environment as well as for your body. Over-fishing is now seen by marine scientists as the single greatest threat to marine wildlife and our oceans. Many fish stocks are in a state of serious decline, with some common stocks on the verge of collapse. The Marine Conservation Society UK has put together a list of the fish from all over the world that appear to be in immediate danger. They include Atlantic cod and Atlantic salmon, as well as snapper, swordfish and tuna (unless it's skipjack tuna, and caught using a pole and line rather than nets). Try to buy fish that is caught at sustainable levels, such as Pacific, or organically farmed, salmon; flounder; Dover and lemon sole; and Pacific cod.

ANOTHER STEP – SUPPLEMENTS

The body needs a wealth of vitamins and minerals to function at optimum levels. Although pure foods can – and should – give us everything we need, sometimes (perhaps when we are exhausted or ill) we need an extra boost in the form of supplements.

Our changing nutritional needs

We are all individuals and we all have different nutritional needs. Age is an important factor – for example, children need many more fats and much more protein, calcium and iron than adults; the elderly often lack calcium and vitamin B12 – but gender, weight, stress levels, overall state of health, levels of physical activity, whether or not you are taking any medication, and even whether or not you smoke and how much alcohol you drink will all influence your specific nutritional needs. The most important nutrients are the four macronutrients (the basic nutrients that we need in large doses: water, carbohydrates, proteins and fats), the micronutrients (the nutrients we need in small doses, but that are nevertheless essential to health: vitamins, minerals and good bacteria; see p.14), and phytonutrients, which we get from plant foods. Ideally, we would receive all these nutrients in just the right quantities from our food. But life is never that simple, right?

Why do we need to take supplements?

The modern diet is largely ill equipped to supply us with all of the nutrients the body requires to maintain optimum health. As we already know, modern farming methods, food-processing and -packaging, transportation times and the way we cook food when we get it home can strip food of its health-giving properties. Although pure foods go some way to redress this balance some sources estimate that less than 5 per cent of the world's population eats a diet rich enough in nutrients and diverse enough in its content to need no supplementation at all. That's not to say that we should switch to supplements and not worry about the nutrient content of our food! I want you to read this book and to come away maximizing the nutritional properties of your food, but also to be unafraid to take supplements sensibly and knowledgeably to make sure that you maintain optimum health.

How to take supplements

HOW MUCH SHOULD I TAKE? Most government food agencies offer guidelines on the RDA (recommended daily amount; also known as RDI – recommended daily intake) for every nutrient. This figure represents the minimum, overall intake of that nutrient in your diet each day to prevent a deficiency – whether you get the nutrient from your food or a supplement, or a combination of both. RDAs are there partly to protect you from any negative side-effects of having too much of a particular nutrient in your system (for example, too much vitamin C, calcium or iron may cause diarrhea or abdominal pain), but actually in most cases the figures are way below the *optimum* daily intake of a supplement – that is, the level that optimizes health. So, unless you have been instructed otherwise by a naturopath or doctor who knows about you and your health, follow the guidelines given in this book (I have listed relevant supplements in each of the plans, and on page 205 given guidelines for the supplements that you may like to take to keep yourself generally fit and young). If you are at all unsure about the suitability of any supplement or its dosage, or if you do experience side-effects, consult a naturopath. Happily, many side-effects will cease once you lower the dosage or stop taking the supplement altogether.

WHEN TO TAKE SUPPLEMENTS The best time to take most supplements is with food, when your digestive tract is most geared up to absorb nutrients into your system. However, probiotics (the "healthy" bacteria) are best taken away from meals, as this improves their chances of surviving the difficult, acidic journey through your stomach.

HOW CLEAN IS OUR WATER?

You are roughly 70 per cent water. This fact alone should give you some idea of just how important water is to your body and so to your overall health. Clean water is also essential to a clean diet.

Clear and clean?

The search for fresh water is a huge daily task in many of the poorer countries on our planet. However, hopefully you simply turn on your tap each day and are guaranteed a supply of something that is both clear and fresh. Note that I use the word "clear" and not necessarily "clean".

We take the safety of our drinking water for granted. Recently, however, naturopaths, doctors and the media have highlighted the dangers of ground-water pollution and some of the health risks from lead, chlorine, pesticides and various micro-organisms that have been found to contaminate municipal water supplies. Outbreaks of waterborne diseases are now common in Western countries and there is growing concern about the potential carcinogenic effects of certain organic chemicals in our water.

What can go wrong?

LEAD CONTAMINATION The heavy metal lead enters our water supplies from the corrosion of water pipes, joint solders in pipes, and plumbing fixtures. Lead in drinking water contributes up to 20 per cent of our total environmental exposure to lead. Young children and babies are particularly vulnerable to lead poisoning, with even low-dose exposure causing intellectual problems and behaviour disorders in those who are susceptible. However, there are some simple steps you can take to reduce the lead in your drinking water:

- Do not drink hot water from the hot tap, nor use it for cooking – hot water dissolves lead more quickly than cold water
- Do not mix baby milk with hot tapwater – use cooled, once-boiled water
- Run the taps for a while before drinking cold water – the fresh, cold water will not have been sitting in contact with pipes or solder
- Test your tapwater for lead and buy a water filter if the levels are high

GERMS AND MICRO-ORGANISMS Ground water, well water, river water, bottled water and some municipal water can contain dangerous micro-organisms (including coliforms, giardia lamblia and cryptosporidium) that can cause diarrhea and vomiting, especially in those who are weak and vulnerable, such as children and the elderly. In the US it is estimated that close to a million people become ill each year owing to bacterial contamination in water.

CHLORINE AND OTHER CHEMICALS Sewerage run-off, industrial chemical pollution, dirty storm water and contaminated run-off from farms and city streets have severely contaminated our water supplies. By-products of chlorine water treatment, such as trihalomethanes, remain in our drinking water after the water has been treated, and are under urgent investigation as possible carcinogens (they may cause cancer). Legal and illegal chemical dumps leak a toxic cocktail into ground water. Arsenic, rocket fuel and a host of other toxic industrial chemicals contaminate most of the water in the UK and US – and around the world.

WE ARE ALL TAKING THE CONTRACEPTIVE PILL Millions of women take the oral contraceptive pill or hormone replacement therapy (HRT) every day. The hormones in these pills pass through the body relatively intact and end up in the urine, from there into our water system, and eventually into our drinking water. This contamination is beginning to cause concern as it may not only contribute to lower sperm counts in men, but it is also thought by some experts to be the cause of more female fish and deformities in the sex organs of some fish, making it difficult or impossible for them to reproduce.

What do we need to do to drink clean water?

DISTILLED WATER – CLEAR WINNER The best water to drink is steam-distilled water. It contains little or no contaminants and is the safest, cleanest and healthiest water available. It is almost pure H_2O. Some say that distilled water depletes the mineral content in the body, however there is no biochemical basis or evidence for such a claim. Others say that distilled water, unlike mineral water, has none of the beneficial minerals in it. In reality, mineral water provides only tiny amounts of the essential minerals you need for health – and besides, our minerals should come from our food, not our water. Distilled water is definitely my winner. Best of all, home distillation units are readily available and relatively cheap to buy.

WATER FILTERS – A CLEAR SECOND Activated carbon filters remove most of the chlorine in tapwater. They also reduce the levels of trihalomethanes, the potentially carcinogenic by-products of chlorination, as well as some pesticides, including fungicides. The level of filtration will depend on the size and type of the filter, the degree of water pollution, and how often you renew the carbon filter. Remember to replace your filters regularly, so that they remain efficient and don't begin to harbour harmful bacteria.

BOTTLED WATER – LAST PLACE Concern over the quality and safety of tapwater has led many of us to rely almost exclusively on bottled drinking water. However, regulations governing the purity and safety of bottled water are less stringent than those for municipal water supplies in most countries. Bottled water is often contaminated with heavy metals, solvents and bacteria. The carcinogenic chemicals (methylene chloride and vinyl chloride) that can enter the water from the plastic-bottle containers are also a major concern.

HOW CLEAN IS OUR AIR?

We can go without food for probably a month. We can go without water for a week or two. How long can we go without oxygen? Hold your breath and see how long it takes before you are forced to take a breath. One minute? Two? Certainly not more than three. Air, and ideally clean air, is absolutely essential for life.

The main air pollutants

Our air contains a bewildering number of contaminants, among them the smoke from the burned fossil fuels we use to generate our electricity, and the gas and petrol we use to heat our homes and run our cars. The following are some of the main air pollutants that we face today.

BURNING FOSSIL FUELS The biggest source of air pollution comes from the fossil fuel-burning power stations that generate our electricity. We all need to make an effort reduce the amount of energy we use. Turn off appliances at night; turn off your computer, or allow it to access the sleep mode, when you are not using it; keep the temperature down a little in your house; open windows in the summer and use air-conditioning sparingly; take the stairs, not the elevator, when you arrive at your apartment block or office building; and turn off unnecessary lights. Saving power means saving the quality of your life.

HEAVY METALS In high enough concentrations, lead (from paint), mercury (from chemical production) and cadmium (from batteries) all have negative health effects. They leach into the soil and from there into the atmosphere and can damage the brain, the immune system and the nervous system. Some heavy metals are known to be carcinogenic (cancer-causing).

PERSISTENT ORGANIC POLLUTANTS (POPS) These toxic pollutants accumulate in humans and animals because they are not easily broken down by our bodies. They include polychlorinated biphenyls (PCBs, by-products of electricity, and plastic and paint manufacturing, among other things), dioxins and furans (produced by most forms of combustion), and pesticides.

AIRBORNE PARTICLES Traffic, construction work and chemical reactions in the air all cause dust, grit, smoke and biological particles. The fine particles irritate the lungs and can cause death in those with lung and heart disease.

CARBON MONOXIDE (CO) This is a toxic gas emitted by combustion processes and it affects the transport of oxygen in the blood. Carbon monoxide poisoning literally suffocates us by starving the brain of oxygen.

Other significant pollutants include ozone, sulphur dioxide, nitrogen oxide, ammonia and hydrogen fluoride. The list is long, and not good news.

What are the effects on our bodies of unclean air?

All pollution leads to the creation of free radicals in the body. Free radicals are also called "oxidants", and they are some of most dangerous chemicals we can have inside us. Unstable and volatile, free radicals zoom around our body looking for ways to stabilize themselves. They do this by stealing electrons (negatively charged particles) from otherwise perfectly healthy atoms in our cells. Once an atom has lost an electron, the atom itself becomes a free radical, and a cascade effect occurs, until eventually the action of the free radicals destroys whole cells in the body. The way to halt free radicals in their tracks is to "mop them up" with certain vitamins, minerals and plant compounds called antioxidants. Some scientists attribute all disease and ageing to the action of free radicals. Taking a regular supplement containing antioxidants such as vitamin C, vitamin A, zinc and selenium is one way to combat the ravages of pollution in the body. However, undoubtedly the best way to guard ourselves against the effects of pollution is to reduce the amount of pollution we create. Take action now! See the box on the opposite page for some ideas on how you can play your part in creating a healthier environment in which to live.

SOME SOLUTIONS TO A POLLUTED WORLD

LEAVE THE CAR AT HOME The average car emits more than 1,000 different pollutants, and transport is estimated to emit between 20 and 25 per cent of all greenhouse gas emissions. Use public transport whenever possible – take the bus, train, metro, subway, tram or underground; share car journeys to and from work or school. Better still, keep all the engines off and walk whenever you can, especially for short journeys; or use a bicycle – it's good for your health and the environment.

BUY A FOREST Planting trees, lots of trees, might just save us and our planet. Trees provide oxygen and remove carbon dioxide from the air. There are some great organizations that plant trees all around the world. Trees make the perfect gift for a loved one or colleague – and for the environment. So, next time you are stuck for inspiration for a birthday or Christmas gift, buy a tree!

GET SOME CLEANER AIR Try to make sure that you get away into the countryside from time to time. The air at the seaside, or up in the mountains, or in the open country, is charged with healthy negative ions (as opposed to the unhealthy positive ions that pollution creates). Breathe deeply and fill your lungs with some of that cleaner oxygen. If you are not able to get away, find your nearest park or woodland and spend a few precious hours in at least fresher air.

GO CARBON NEUTRAL There is an amazing organization called The CarbonNeutral Company, based in the UK, that helps to reduce the impact businesses have on the environment by working with them to reduce carbon emissions. The organization has a website (see p.229) that is packed with information, as well as products you can buy (from anywhere in the world) that do their bit for the environment.

MAX FACT

In a single day, Southern California's lawnmowers produce more pollution than all the aircraft in the Los Angeles area. A single mower puts out more pollution than 73 modern cars.

HOW TO USE THE DIET PLANS

The chapters in the rest of this book are dedicated to cleaning up your diet using pure foods – here's how to get the best from them.

Choosing the right plan for you

Chapters 2, 3 and 4 present the Detox, Digestion tune-up and Energy-boost plans respectively, each of them divided into three step-by-step programs lasting a weekend, a week and a month. To decide which plan will be of greatest benefit to you, answer the questionnaire opposite – the column with the highest score shows your area (body system) of greatest need. Then decide whether to undertake the relevant plan for a weekend, a week or a month. Guidance on this is given for each plan, on pages 47, 85 and 123 respectively.

At the end of Chapter 4 is a special plan that gives an optimum health cleanse. This Pure-foods Total Cleanse runs together all three of the other plans, so that you go from one plan into the next, without a break, in a total body-system workout. Use the questionnaire to decide which plan to use first (as before), but this time do the plan with the highest score for one month; with the next highest score for a week; and with the lowest score for a weekend.

Use Chapter 5, the Ailment Plans, if you want to alleviate or prevent a specific condition using pure foods; or if you need to boost your immune system. I have given detailed information on 14 major conditions, as well as essential information for a further 15 conditions in the chart on pages 192–3. And finally, Chapter 6 is your maintenance plan. When you feel fit and well, use the advice in this chapter to ensure that you optimize your wellbeing and keep your body fit, young and slim well into your future.

THE CLEAN UP YOUR DIET QUESTIONNAIRE

This questionnaire will help you to identify whether you most need a detox, digestion or energy cleanse. Please take time to read the statements carefully and then mark in pencil those that most apply to you at this time. When you have finished, count up the number of marks you have made in each column. The highest score wins – this is the plan that you should embark upon now. Note that a month from now, your answers may be different, so do keep coming back to the questionnaire from time to time to see if you need a different cleanse. If you are doing the pure-foods total cleanse (p.154), the highest score goes first and gets the month-long treatment. Follow with the one-week plan for the next highest score, and then the weekend for the lowest.

THE DETOX

My breath smells at times

I can have strong body odour

My eyes are red and can itch

I have been drinking a lot of alcohol and coffee/tea/fizzy drinks lately

I feel stiff, slow-moving and old

My hair, skin and nails are in poor condition

I am overweight

I catch a cold very easily

I feel like I am carrying excess fluids; I feel puffy

I need to regain control of my diet and lifestyle

I crave sugary and/or junk foods

I have taken a lot of prescribed antibiotics recently

THE DIGESTIVE TUNE-UP

I feel bloated and full after meals

I feel tired after eating

I am constipated (fewer than six bowel motions a week)

I get regular diarrhea (more often than once a week)

I am flatulent

I burp after eating/food often repeats on me

My tongue is yellowish or coated in the mornings

I do not have a good appetite

I have pains in my stomach or strong discomfort after eating

I often have undigested food in my stool

I have alternating constipation and diarrhea

I seem to be sensitive/allergic to some foods

THE ENERGY-BOOST

I am tired and lethargic

My sex drive is low

I am in desperate need of a holiday but can't take the time off

I don't seem to be able to get enough sleep; I wake unrefreshed

I am sleepy during the day, especially in the afternoon

I wake at night feeling restless

I am irritable and jumpy

I have so much to do and don't feel I can cope

I feel sad or down much of the time

Small things really annoy me

I have trouble concentrating

I need strong stimulants, such as coffee, to make it through my day

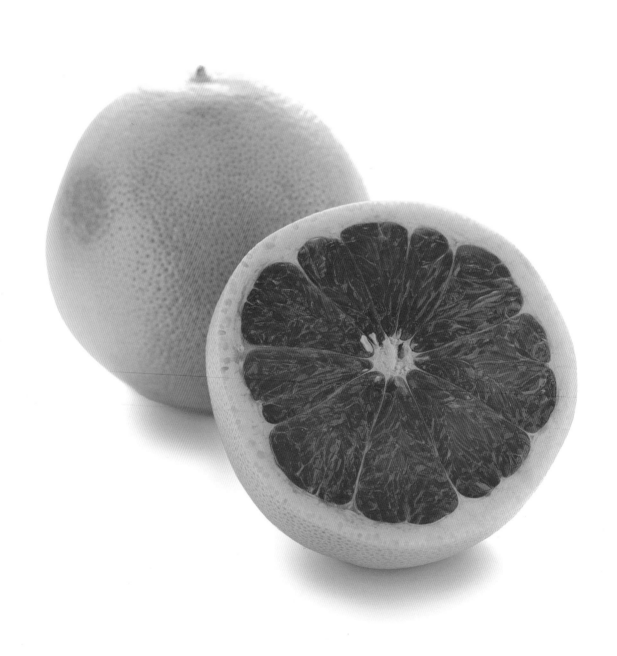

the detox plans

make use of the amazing power of pure foods to detox, heal and lose weight

DO YOU NEED TO CLEAN UP YOUR ACT?

ARE YOU:

Overweight and overfed?

Suffering from constipation or bad breath?

Plagued with lacklustre skin and hair?

Smoking or drinking too much?

Craving chocolates and sweets all the time?

Taking a lot of prescribed conventional medicines?

Worried about acne and oily skin?

Tired of aches and pains in your joints?

Keen to feel cleaner and leaner?

If you answered yes to any these questions, you are most probably suffering from a build-up of toxins and are in need of a pure-foods clean-out. Grab this chance to clean up your body and return to a state of vibrant health. The work is hard, but the rewards are amazing.

WHAT IS DETOX?

Detox, a wonderful, geniune naturopathic term, has become an overused "buzz word", the darling of the glossy magazines and the icon of a new form of preventive medicine. It is a word most often used with no understanding of the real healing it offers. I want to give you a clear picture of what it means to be toxic and then show you how to clean up your act with pure foods.

The importance of detox

Naturopaths are clear that the elimination of toxins through detoxing is the key to good health. What goes into the body in the form of food, air and water, must be used by the body to promote health and vitality – otherwise the body must eliminate it. Anything that the body does not eliminate, accumulates. You then become toxic. Fact. From a naturopathic perspective this is one of the main causes of disease. If your food, air and water are polluted by chemicals, the need to eliminate effectively becomes a major priority in the maintenance of health. If we add to this the fact that your own body produces toxins as a by-product of metabolism, stress and exercise, you have a good case for needing a strong system of elimination.

How are we exposed to toxins?

We all live in a polluted world. Each day we take in a nasty array of chemicals with our food and drink and the air we breathe. The list is long and really quite scary: exhaust fumes; insecticides and pesticides; food preservatives, colourings, flavourings, thickeners and enhancers; and chemical pollution and industrial pollution are all major culprits. However, for millions of

"Modern chemical production has given our bodies a vast array of unnatural, manmade chemicals to deal with. We are in the middle of a chemical war."

years, as our bodies developed, we were exposed to a fairly narrow range of natural chemicals. Our bodies knew how to deal with these and so very few of the natural chemicals actually accumulated in our tissues and caused damage to our health. The situation now is altogether different.

Most modern farm chemicals have side-effects and are a good example of the toxins we have to deal with in today's world. For example, pesticides, such as organophosphates and organochlorines, can cause a whole range of side-effects including headaches, dizziness, weakness, shaking, nausea, stomach cramps, diarrhea, sweating, rashes, loss of appetite, weight loss, disorientation, nervousness and a general feeling of illness. Another good example is instant coffee – most brands contain more than 1,000 chemicals, some of which scientists have shown to cause cancer in mice. If these damaging chemical toxins are not eliminated effectively from our bodies, we become toxic and suffer a greater chance of falling ill by one means or another.

How can toxins damage us?

If your body is toxic, you will experience a range of problems. These often present warning signs showing you that it's time to detox.

TOXINS AND FLUCTUATING WEIGHT The body stores uneliminated toxins in body fat, because the fat depot tends to be stable and so does not often break down and release its toxic load into the blood and other tissues (unless we lose a lot of weight). Our wonderful, clever bodies also hold on to excess water to dilute the toxins, creating water retention. So, the more toxic you are, the more weight you gain – and retain!

TOXINS AND HORMONE IMBALANCES Some insecticides and pesticides mimic the action of our own hormones, which are important natural body chemicals and include estrogen, progesterone and adrenaline (epinephrine). Hormones run essential functions, such as reproduction, energy production and blood-sugar management. Farm chemicals are so close to our natural hormones in structure that they create hormone imbalances in us, leading to problems with the management of many of our essential body processes.

TOXINS AND DAMAGE TO YOUR BODY'S CELLS The most significant damage happens at an atomic level. The basic components of all matter are known as atoms and they consist of a nucleus of protons and neutrons surrounded by electrons. An atom that has lost an electron is known as a free radical. I know that we've mentioned the free radical before, but, to recap, it

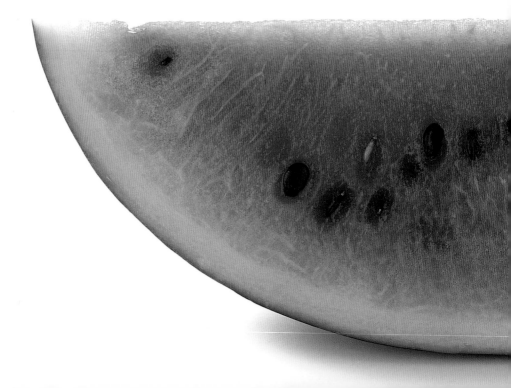

will stop at nothing in its quest to steal an electron and complete itself. In the process it degrades natural body chemicals, disrupts internal biochemistry and creates disease. Scientists have directly linked free radicals with diseases ranging from cancer to arthritis and tell us that they are created by common factors such as stress, but also by toxins, such as environmental pollution and poor food. Heated oils, rancid oils and too much alcohol all create free radicals. The only protection you have against these little horrors is a group of natural chemicals found in abundance in pure foods – the free-radical killing antioxidants, such as vitamin C and the mineral selenium.

How do we eliminate?

The major routes of elimination in your body are your lungs, your liver, your bowels (via the stool), your skin and your kidneys (via urine). In other words, nature has supplied your body with a variety of effective routes for getting rid of toxins. However, for most of us, the elimination pathways are permanently overloaded and so under immense strain.

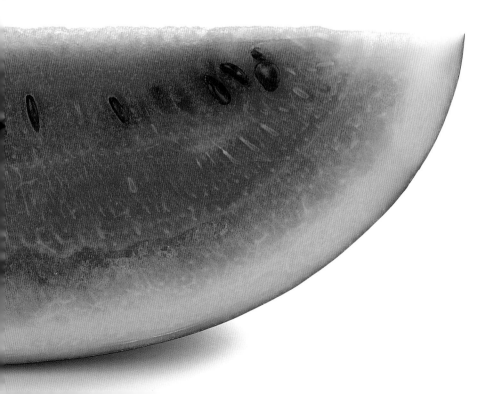

WHY ARE THE ELIMINATION PATHWAYS IN TROUBLE?

Your lungs may be overloaded with cigarette smoke, air-borne pollution and a general lack of fresh air and exercise. Your liver may have to deal with fatty diets, manmade chemicals, high alcohol consumption and a vast array of prescription and recreational drugs. Your bowels are often constipated and thus accumulate waste instead of eliminating it. Your poor kidneys are often starved of water to flush out toxins and your skin does not see cleansing sunshine or regular exfoliation. Another major problem is what naturopaths call "enervation", or low nervous energy. Simply put, your nervous system governs and controls the systems and organs of elimination and in many people it is tired and just not up to the job. Stress, busy schedules, late nights and myriad other commitments modern living throws at you have exhausted your poor nervous system. A tired you is a toxic you.

Switching to pure foods

Detoxing is all about giving your body a rest from the strain that life puts on it – and that begins by cleaning up your diet. The idea is that by reducing the amount of sifting your body has to do before it begins the process of assimilating and digesting nutrients, you will have more energy for getting the most out of your food, which in turn means that your overall energy levels and your health improve. If you are overweight, you will also begin to lose weight.

Turning to organic foods (or at least washing all your fruits and vegetables thoroughly; your local health-food store will probably stock a special wash) will hugely decrease the load on your systems of elimination by the simple fact that you are saving them from having to deal with a host of chemical fertilizers. The fact that pure foods contain no nasty chemical additives, in the forms of colourings, flavourings, preservatives, enhancers and so on, compounds this overall lightening of the toxic load. The final thing worth a special mention is that pure foods are rich in two particularly crucial detox nutrients. These nutrients are antioxidants, which zip about your body mopping up all the disease-causing free radicals (see pp.44–5), and fibre, which helps to ensure that you open and empty your bowels (your body's waste-disposal unit) every day, so that the toxins in your stool are not reabsorbed into your body, which would make the toxic overload even worse.

How the detox plans work

Over the following pages you will find the three detox plans – one that lasts for a weekend (see pp.52–5), one that lasts for a week (see pp.58–60) and a final plan that lasts for a month (see pp.61–3). By completing the questionnaire on page 39, you have already decided that your systems of elimination most need some help and you need to detox; now you need to decide which of the three specific detox plans is best suited to you.

WHICH PLAN SHOULD I USE – WEEKEND, WEEK OR MONTH?

I recommend the weekend detox if you are completely new to detoxing – it will gently introduce you to the amazing effect that detox can have on how you feel, and will almost certainly inspire you to progress to the longer detoxes (immediately or next time). The weekend plan is also great if you are a regular detoxer who just needs a quick top-up, perhaps after a heavy week. If you have had a sustained period of indulgence or have been on antibiotics (and are now well), the week- or month-long detoxes will be best for you. The most crucial thing is to embark on the plan that you will see through to the end – it's important for your mental wellbeing that you complete what you set out to do.

HOW ARE THE PLANS LAID OUT?

Each plan is divided into three steps. The first step, Preparation, shows you how to prepare for the time ahead so that you are motivated and focused on your detox. Step two is the Menu Plan, which gives you information about the meals that you will eat and refers you directly to the relevant recipes on pages 64–77. I urge you to stick to the menu plan throughout your detox as it will ensure that you maximize your intake of the nutrients appropriate for reducing the load on your systems of elimination and cleansing you right through. Finally, detoxing is as much about cleaning up your lifestyle as it is about clean food. A frantic or stressful lifestyle is not going to make for a good detox – you will be too exhausted to get the best out of the process. A completely sedentary lifestyle is just as bad. A balance between activity and rest ensures a plentiful supply of the energy you need to undertake a cleanse. Regular exercise and stretching keep your body in shape, while a daily relaxation helps to maintain emotional wellbeing while you clean out. Step three (Action) in each of the detoxes will guide you on exactly what to do.

INTRODUCING THE DETOX PLANS

These detox plans are the first steps on the journey to a leaner, cleaner, healthier you. Over the past 20 years, I have helped thousands of my clients to detox. It need not be elaborate or difficult – all you need are some pure foods and motivation.

The benefits of the detox plans

The general aim is a "leaner and cleaner" you. The detox plans reduce the load on your organs of elimination by reducing your overall intake of toxins, giving you a chance to clean up and feel great. The specific health benefits include a reduction in your intake of synthetic chemicals (including pesticides and insecticides), an increase in protective antioxidants, and a marked improvement in immune function. You should also notice an increase in energy, better sleep patterns and an improvement in skin tone and texture. Obviously, the benefits are greater the longer you persevere. Begin at the weekend – and keep going!

General rules for the detox plans

SAY NO TO DRUGS! This means alcohol, caffeine, nicotine and other recreational drugs – they place a huge strain on your elimination system. (Never stop taking prescribed medication without consulting your doctor.)

CUT OUT THE IMMUNITY ENEMIES This includes all sugar products, such as condiments, cakes, pastries, candy, and so on; and all allergens, such as wheat, and cow's dairy. Both these groups of food depress the immune system, which is responsible for identifying and helping to eliminate toxins through the lymph. Too much sugar or too many allergenic foods simply leave you at risk of keeping more toxins in your blood. If you need sweetness, add some organic honey or rice malt to your foods. (See page 87 for substituting allergens.)

CUT OUT THE JUNK AND FRIED FOODS Junk foods include all packaged, tinned and processed foods, many of which contain harmful chemicals and additives. Tinned foods may also leach metal compounds into their contents, which may be damaging to your health. Apart from being cooked with additive-laden commercial oils, fried foods are often more likely to harbour harmful free radicals, as oil turns rancid and unstable as it heats up. Steaming, baking and grilling (broiling) are suitable ways to cook during a detox; and of course eat as many raw foods as you can.

EAT ORGANIC MEAT AND FISH Although fish is often seen as the healthy option, according to some sources, more than 80 per cent of swordfish, for example, are contaminated with mercury, and more than 40 per cent of salmon contain traces of PCBs (polychlorinated biphenyls – a manmade oily chemical). Non-organic meat and poultry may be fattened up using chemical antibiotics (see pp.16–17). All this adds to the strain on your elimination organs.

DRINK 2 LITRES (4 PINTS) OF WATER A DAY Water helps to flush out your system, keeping your kidneys working at their optimum levels. Make the water distilled or carbon-filtered (see p.34), and add a squeeze of lemon juice to it, as this helps to stimulate liver function. Drink your water at room temperature as this is better for your stomach and bowels, and try to drink it away from mealtimes so as not to dilute your digestive juices (see p.87).

REDUCE YOUR SALT INTAKE Salt impairs the movement of fluids through the tissues of the body – especially through the lymphatic system, which is a major route for the elimination of toxins.

In addition, try to practise food combining in the evenings; try not to eat after 8pm; and try to make lunch your biggest meal of the day (see pp.86–7). All these things will help you to feel and become leaner and lighter.

Side-effects during the plans

If you are a caffeine-user (that is, you drink coffee, tea or caffeine-loaded fizzy drinks), you might experience headaches as you withdraw from this stimulant. Use the homeopathic Coffea 6X or C to help reduce the severity of the headaches if they are really bad. I suggest taking two pillules under the tongue up to four times a day. Suck them and try to relax and breathe deeply. The increased intake of fruits and vegetables could cause you to feel quite bloated for the first few days. Chop your salads finely so that they are easier for your gut to handle, chew well, and take a digestive enzyme supplement containing cellulase (see opposite) to keep bloating to a minimum.

Do not be surprised if you experience any of the following on the longer cleanses: minor diarrhea, runny nose, nausea, sore throat, acne, bad breath, or mild fever. These are just the normal signs that your body is enjoying a clean-out – in natural medicine we call them healing crises. Most will pass in a day or two. Just stick to the program and let your body do its work.

What's on the menu?

None of my plans is a fast! There are three meals every day, each one brimming with pure-food nutrients. Most importantly, by drinking a pure fruit smoothie or juice every morning, having fruit for breakfast on most days and eating fruit as your dessert at dinnertime, you will dramatically boost your intake of

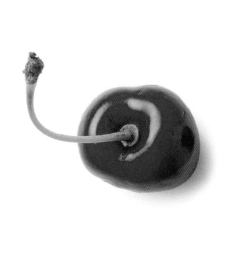
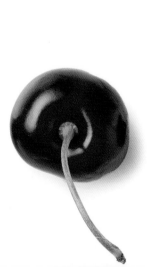
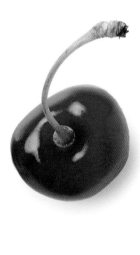

antioxidants (see p.45) and, crucially, fibre, which will get your bowels working. I've tried to include plenty of spices, especially ginger, which helps to boost your circulation and lymphatic system and literally "sweat out" toxins through the skin. Most of the recipes in this chapter are dairy-, wheat- and/or gluten-free to reduce the allergenic load (see pp.48–9).

First-aid detox supplements

The following are the supplements that will help to maximize elimination.

- Milk thistle helps to motivate the liver to break down fats. I suggest using a fresh plant tincture (liquid). Take it according to the bottle instructions.
- Chromium polynicotinate (400mcg a day) will stabilize blood sugars and reduce any hunger pangs and sugar cravings.
- Digestive enzymes (find a formula containing protease, lipase, amylase, cellulose, phytase, lactase, sucrase and maltase) will help to calm digestion and inhibit any bloating. Take one with each meal during a detox.
- A probiotic with lactobacillus acidophilus and bifidus ("good" bacteria) promotes good digestion and keeps bad bacteria under control in the gut.
- Essential fatty acids aid digestion, weight-loss, and blood-sugar and hormone balance. Take a balanced formula containing omega-3, -6 and -9.
- Take a "green" drink containing raw, dried organic greens such as chlorella, spirulina, alfalfa, barley, rye, broccoli, parsley and kale. Greens provide us with fibre and plant nutrients, and are the best sources of antioxidants.

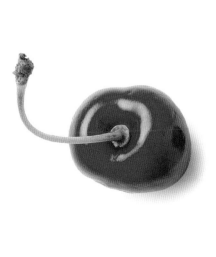
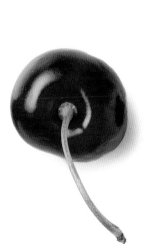
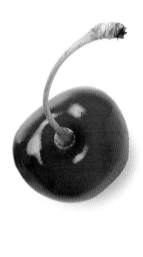

INTRODUCING THE WEEKEND DETOX

Anyone should be able to do the weekend detox plan – it's just 48 short hours out of your life; but the impact on your body is much longer lasting. This is the place to begin.

Why should I do the weekend plan?

The weekend detox gives your liver, bowels and kidneys a much-needed rest and allows these valuable organs to do two full days of house cleaning. Your increased intake of distilled or filtered water and of Max's detox herbal tea (see opposite) will initiate a deep cleanse by stimulating your lymphatic system to drain toxins away from your cells. The abundance of vitamins and minerals in pure foods will flood into the blood stream and wash over your cells, providing the nutrients you need to maintain health at a deep, cellular level. The increased intake of protective antioxidants will neutralize active free radicals and help to undo some of the damage done by your past free-radical load.

What benefits will I see and feel?

The most tangible overall benefit will be an improvement in your appearance, particularly in your skin tone and the sparkle in your eyes; but the very first benefit has to be a sense of calm anticipation that settles over your body as you take the first steps toward a weekend of detoxing. By skipping your morning coffee or tea, you give yourself the chance to wake slowly, naturally, instead of your usual morning ritual of "stop" to "full-throttle" in a split, caffeine-fuelled second. By the second stimulant-free morning, you will start to feel your natural energy coming through. Supplement it with a good stretch and some breathing. Your bowels will start to quieten down as you remove the foods that normally bloat you (bread, pasta, sugar and so on) and, if you are taking it, the digestive enzyme (see p.51) improves your ability to break down your food. You may find that you have a full bowel motion for the first time in ages as the increased fibre and fluids in your fruits and vegetables takes effect.

Finishing the detox plans

Give yourself a little extra push and finish your detox on Monday morning, rather than Sunday night. When you've finished you will feel cleaner, leaner and fresher, but you might also feel a bit wobbly (especially when you finish the longer plans) and will perhaps need to reintroduce yourself to the world gently. Bring back non-detox foods slowly, as this allows you to gauge if they do not agree with you (particularly, cow's dairy and wheat). If you get bloated or tired after eating a particular food, just keep it out of your diet for a bit longer. Try to avoid going back to refined white-flour products, such as white bread and pasta; simple sugars, such as those found in cakes and sweets; and fatty, fried foods. Were you surprised that you could survive without coffee and tea? Think hard before bringing back any stimulants. You do not need them – they give you a false sense of wellbeing and will exhaust you in the long term.

Finally, try to make a habit of some of the elements of the detox. Start your day with a cleansing smoothie, commit to regular exercise and say no to one naughty snack each day. Stretch to keep your spine, joints and muscles young. Then, plan to do a regular top-up detox every three months. Do just a quick weekend refresher to remind you how good it feels to be clean on the inside.

MAX'S DETOX HERBAL TEA

To prepare the dried tea, mix together equal parts of these dried, organic herbs: pau d'arco, mullein, red clover, yellow dock, dandelion root (chopped), burdock root and milk thistle seed.

When you are ready to make the tea, place a teaspoon of the dried herb mix per cup into a tea pot. Allow the tea to steep in boiling water for five minutes, then pour. Add fresh, grated lemon peel and ginger root to taste. Drink and enjoy!

THE WEEKEND DETOX PLAN

Step 1: preparation

A good cleanse needs a little planning. It would be a tragedy if you got all the way to Sunday afternoon only to succumb to that chocolate biscuit hiding in the cupboard. Solution? Clear your cupboards and your refrigerator of anything that you know in your heart is a poor food. Crisps, biscuits, cakes, oven chips, burger buns, and tinned custard have got to go. Remove all of the temptations so that you can focus on your detox.

Clean the house on Thursday night. Wash your sheets and air your bedroom so that you have a fabulous, clean bed to jump into on Friday. Make sure you have all your favourite clothes clean, especially some comfortable baggy pants and your favourite T-shirt. You are going to be a bit of a hermit this weekend so dress comfortably. The only time you'll leave the house will be to have a brisk walk in the fresh air.

Make sure you have all the props you need for a weekend of peace. Get some magazines and a few movies and make sure you have some candles to set the mood in your bathroom and bedroom. Turn off your cellphone and put on your answerphone.

A SPECIAL NOTE ABOUT BREAKFAST It is vital during the detox to start your day on the right note. Your body has been cleaning and detoxing during the night and so breakfast should facilitate this process. A good, healthy breakfast of pure foods helps the body to continue to clean out.

Step 2: menu plan

DAY ONE

Cleanse:aid smoothie (first thing in the morning) Cleansing cocktail (p.68)

Breakfast Berry fruit salad (p.64)

Lunch Persian rice with tomato saffron sauce (p.70)

Dinner Roast salmon and beetroot (beet) salad (p.74); and for dessert a piece of fresh fruit eaten half an hour after your main course

Before bed Max's detox herbal tea (p.53)

DAY TWO

Cleanse:aid juice Hot lemon and ginger (p.66)

Breakfast Berry fruit salad (p.64)

Lunch Ginger chicken skewers with quinoa tabbouleh (p.72)

Dinner Three-bean chilli with avocado salsa (p.75); and for dessert a piece of fresh fruit eaten half an hour after your main course

Before bed Max's detox herbal tea (p.53)

SNACKS AND SMOOTHIES
Snacks are not banned on the detox, but restrict them to fresh fruit, raw vegetables, raw nuts, and seeds (such as sunflower and pumpkin seeds). Keep near you a small airtight container filled with vegetable crudités (such as cucumber, celery and apples), so that you always have something healthy to snack on. Try to drink at least one additional health-giving juice or smoothie (see pp.66–9) each day.

Step 3: action

Aim to do 15 to 20 minutes of Breathing, Relaxing, Stretching (BRS) each day during the detox. Use the exercises in Chapter 6 too.

BREATHING Oxygen energizes the mind and body and helps to burn off toxins, neutralizing them through a process called oxidation, and preparing them for elimination. Spend a few minutes each morning in front of an open window, inhaling air deeply into your lungs.

RELAXING Stress robs the nervous system of energy and this in turn retards its ability to oversee the elimination of toxins. There is a difference between true relaxation (yoga, a deep bath, meditation and so on) and "participation" (such as dinner with friends, or a movie show). True relaxation leaves you with a renewed sense of wellbeing, charged up for the detox. Schedule in some form of relaxation each day. I suggest a long bath or a walk in the park. If at any point the detox makes you feel edgy (this is quite normal), practise the whole body relaxation on the right.

STRETCHING Prepare your mind and body for the day by gently practising the following stretch to wake up your body. In particular the stretch opens up the chest, helping you to breathe more effectively. Stand with your feet wide apart and breathe in. Raise your arms straight up and lock your fingers. Moving from your waist, bend the body first to the right and then to the left, exhaling as you bend and inhaling as you come back to the upright position. Repeat five times on each side.

WHOLE BODY RELAXATION

1 Find a comfortable position, either on the floor or in a chair. Dim the lighting. Take three deep breaths, breathing right down into your stomach. Breathe in relaxation through the nose, and breathe out all your tension through the mouth.

2 Bring your awareness to your right foot. Visualize your big toe, and relax it. Do the same with each right toe in turn – slowly and gently. Continue up your right leg, visualizing each part in turn then relaxing it to let the tension go. Do this slowly and purposefully. Don't hurry. Visualize the sole of your right foot, then the top of the foot, the ankle, shin, calf, knee, front of the thigh, back of the thigh, and right buttock. The whole right leg is warm and relaxed. Repeat on your left foot and leg. Slowly.

3 Imagine, and consciously relax, both buttocks; then slowly your lower back, mid back, space between the shoulder blades, shoulders, neck, scalp, forehead, space between the eyebrows, eyebrows, eyes, eyelids, nose and nostrils, mouth, tongue, jaw, cheeks, chin, and head. Your neck, shoulders, face and head are now fully relaxed and warm.

4 Slowly move on to visualize and consciously relax your chest, upper abdomen, lower abdomen and pelvis. Now visualize and try to consciously relax all your internal organs – your heart, spleen, liver, kidneys and so on.

5 Bring your awareness to your right arm. Relax the fingers, palm of the hand, wrist, forearm, elbow, upper arm, and shoulder. Your whole right arm is relaxed and warm. Repeat on your left arm.

6 Your whole body is relaxed and warm. Enjoy the sense of peace. Imagine all your internal organs functioning perfectly, removing toxins from your blood and tissues. You feel cleaner, lighter, healthier.

THE DEEPER DETOX

Fabulous! You've done the weekend plan and now you're going to keep going for five more days, or even another three weeks! I could not be happier – this is where the long-term benefits really begin.

Why should I choose a longer detox?

With your newfound sense of wellbeing you are just so ready to take on a full week – or even a full four weeks – so that you can "detox to the Max"! The new, focused you is totally ready for this next step. During the longer plans, your appearance should undergo fairly major changes as your skin's colour and texture improve. (The skin suffers when you are toxic, as nutrients that are important for skin health are redirected to other parts of the body to combat the toxicity.) You should notice a gradual reduction in weight and a firming up of your tissues as excess fluids are mopped up and excreted. Detoxing tends to clear up any digestive problems, reducing abdominal bloating and the primary symptom of digestive problems – smelly breath.

Temptation and treats

Temptation – a quick cup of coffee, or a tasty chocolate – will creep up on you during your extended detox. My favourite temptation-buster is distraction. Leave the kitchen or the café immediately and focus on this little mental mantra – say to yourself: "It's bad for me, it makes me toxic." Feel the words and remember why you started the detox in the first place. If this fails the next option is to phone or text a friend with a pre-arranged cry for help. The craving or temptation should be gone by the time your wise friend returns your call or text with kind words of admonishment.

As for treats, I accept that four weeks is a long time to go without any treats at all! Try to restrict treats to fresh fruit, raw nuts, seeds, and, best of all, non-food treats such as a visit to a gallery or a musical. You are also allowed the treat of a delicious fruit dessert – the only rule that applies to this is to wait half an hour after dinner before tucking in. This allows your dinner to settle first.

Deeper detoxes and everyday life

Longer detoxes will inevitably conflict with your normal daily routine. Ask friends, colleagues and family to work around you for the weeks that you are detoxing. You may not feel like doing your duty at times (you might feel a bit under the weather), so ask others to help with routine things, such as picking up the kids from school or doing the grocery shopping. If you are the one who cooks for your family, ask everyone else to eat what you are eating.

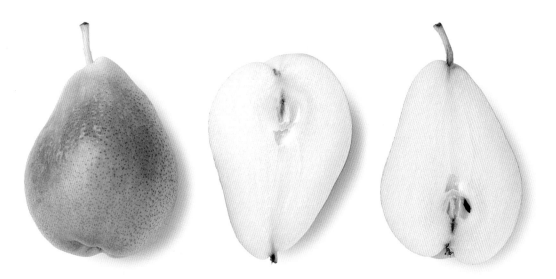

MAX'S MOTIVATOR

Visualize yourself looking and feeling great at the end of your detox program. Close your eyes and imagine yourself in your favourite clothes looking in the mirror. See how clear your skin is and how much healthier and fitter you look and feel. Do this whenever the going gets tough.

THE ONE-WEEK DETOX PLAN

Step 1: preparation

The weekend detox (pp.54–5) provides you with days one and two of your week-long (seven-day) plan. Here you'll find guidance for days three to seven. Once you've done the weekend, you will have done all the hard work, but can I now ask you to get rid of all the synthetic cleaning chemicals in your house? Replace them with eco-friendly products. Visit your local health-food store and find a range made from natural products, such as vinegar, lemon juice and essential oils. I use them in my home and it is nice and clean!

If you are at work, clear your diary of all but essential meetings so that you can keep your head down, do your job and focus on detoxing. Incorporate a healthy walk part of the way to work rather than taking the bus, car or train the whole way. Warn your friends and family about the detox and ask them to keep food and drink temptations out of your way. Take a look at the recipes for the week and do all your shopping in one go. Missing ingredients can really spoil a recipe and will make it easier to substitute non-detox foods.

I always find that some form of inspirational reading can work wonders when you need a lift. For me it's reading about the philosophy of natural medicine, but *The Prophet* by Kahil Gibran or any of Paul Coelho's books are great if you are feeling concerned about committing to an extended detox.

Step 2: menu plan

I think you always suspected that food was hugely important for the maintenance of health. Now you know it is. After a few days on pure foods you have already started to notice the difference to your sleep, the colour of your skin and the efficiency of your bowels. One word of warning though. If you have traditionally been a vegetable-shy human being, preferring to push anything green, white or red to the side of your plate, you are in for a nasty surprise. You are eating a lot more plant fibre at the moment and this can lead to ... how shall I put it politely? Flatulence on a grand scale. The reason for this is that plant fibre – known as cellulose – is extremely hard for us to digest and we need to have certain bacteria in the gut to help us. It takes time for your body to cultivate the correct bacteria, and your stomach and bowels need to make other small adjustments to your digestion process before things can calm down. Please don't give up and, if it gets really bad, I suggest getting down to your local health-food store to buy some digestive enzymes, exactly as I recommend in the supplements section on p.51. They will help to break down the fibres and calm the bloating.

NOTE: In the following menu plan, use days one and two from the Weekend Detox Plan. Turn to page 60 for Step 3: action of the one-week plan.

ONE-WEEK MENU PLAN

DAY 3

Detox:aid juice (for first thing in the morning) Hot lemon and ginger (p.66)

Breakfast Berry fruit salad (p.64)

Lunch Refreshing watermelon salad (p.71)

Dinner Really red risotto (p.74); and for dessert eat a piece of fresh fruit half an hour after your main course

Before bed Max's detox herbal tea (p.53)

DAY 4

Cleanse:aid smoothie (for first thing in the morning) Cleansing cocktail (p.68)

Breakfast Green fruit salad (p.64)

Lunch Garlic grilled (broiled) sardines with pomegranate salsa (p.71)

Dinner Chicken Waldorf salad (p.73); and for dessert eat a piece of fresh fruit half an hour after your main course

Before bed Max's detox herbal tea (p.53)

DAY 5

Detox:aid juice (for first thing in the morning) Hot lemon and ginger (p.66)

Breakfast Egg on toast (p.65)

Lunch Soup au pistou (p.72)

Dinner Griddled tuna with Italian five-bean salad (p.73); and for dessert eat a piece of fresh fruit half an hour after your main course

Before bed Max's detox herbal tea (p.53)

DAY 6

Cleanse:aid smoothie (for first thing in the morning) Cleansing cocktail (p.68)

Breakfast Max's muesli (p.65)

Lunch Persian rice with tomato saffron risotto (p.70)

Dinner Roast salmon and beetroot (beet) salad (p.74); and for dessert eat a piece of fresh fruit half an hour after your main course

Before bed Max's detox herbal tea (p.53)

DAY 7

Detox:aid juice (for first thing in the morning) Hot lemon and ginger (p.66)

Breakfast Berry fruit salad (p.64)

Lunch Ginger chicken skewers with quinoa tabbouleh (p.72)

Dinner Three-bean chilli with avocado salsa (p.75); and for dessert eat a piece of fresh fruit half an hour after your main course

Before bed Max's detox herbal tea (p.53)

SNACKS AND SMOOTHIES

As with the weekend detox, please restrict snacks to fresh fruit, raw vegetables, raw nuts, and seeds (such as sunflower and pumpkin). Keep a small, airtight container of fruit or vegetable crudités (cucumber, celery and apples are ideal) near you, so that you always have something healthy to snack on. If you are hungry after breakfast, have a small handful of mixed nuts and seeds. Try to drink at least one other detox juice or smoothie (see pp.66–9) every day.

Step 3: action

Feel free to adjust the following Breathing, Relaxing, Stretching (BRS) schedule to suit your lifestyle. Aim to do 20–30 minutes BRS each day.

BREATHING This technique teaches you to focus on your breathing. By breathing deeply you will aid the elimination of toxins from your lungs. Sit in a comfortable position with your back straight and your head tilted slightly forward. Close your eyes and take a few deep breaths. Let your breath flow naturally – don't force it; it should be quiet, slow and easy. Now count "1" as you exhale. The next time you exhale count "2", then "3" and so on up to "5". On the next exhalation, begin a new cycle by counting "1" again. Keep counting your exhalations in cycles of 5 for 10 minutes. You will know your attention has wandered away from the breath when you find yourself counting higher than "5"! Practise this exercise once or twice a day.

RELAXING It is easier to focus on the detox if you are mentally calm and physically relaxed. Try to do the cleansing light visualization (right) every day; it builds on the relaxation you did over the weekend.

STRETCHING This stretch helps to massage your bowels. Lie flat on your back. Bend your right leg and bring your thigh toward your chest. Interlock your fingers and place them over your knee. Inhale deeply and exhale, emptying your lungs as much as possible. Without inhaling, lift your head and chest and try to touch your right knee with your nose. Inhale slowly and return to a lying position. Do the stretch 10 times altogether and then change legs.

CLEANSING LIGHT VISUALIZATION

1 Begin with the relaxation you have been practising over the weekend. When you have finished say to yourself: "My whole body is relaxed and warm; my whole body is relaxed and warm."

2 Picture two taps in the soles of your feet. Open these taps and allow all of your negativity to flood out of them. Gather together all your pain, discomfort, disappointment, anger and frustration and imagine them all flooding out as a dark, foul-smelling liquid. You are letting go of all the toxins in your body. Send the stream of liquid directly upward and into the sun to be burned.

3 Feel the cool air entering your nostrils, and the warm air leaving. Focus on this for a few breaths. Imagine now that you are breathing in the light of health. This is a golden light that enters the body through the nostrils.

4 Feel the light seeping into the mind, clearing and cleansing. Feel the light moving downward through your body, pushing the darkness before it. It moves to your shoulders, down through your chest and abdomen, into both your legs and down to the taps in your feet. Where there is light there can be no dark. Where there is health there can be no disease.

5 Now that the light has moved down through your body to the taps, you have pushed all the darkness away so that there is light entering through your nostrils and exiting through the taps in your feet. Your body is cleansed. Your body is purified. Close the taps and feel the warmth in your body. Lie or sit still for a few moments and then get up slowly.

EXTENDING THE PLAN TO FOUR WEEKS

Congratulations on completing the one-week plan! Now it's time to do something truly remarkable for your body and make the commitment to the four-week detox plan. Every day will build on your achievements so far until you feel entirely like new.

Preparing, Eating and BRS

The week-long detox has given you all the preparation you need for another three weeks – just don't forget to top up the shopping. The eating schedule for the next three weeks is set out for you on pages 62–3. As far as Breathing, Relaxing, Stretching is concerned, the four-week plan simply combines the techniques you've already learned. Open your windows wide each morning and breathe deeply; use the more meditative "count your breath" technique (see p.60) at night, not only to enhance your breathing but also to calm you before sleep. Do the stretch on page 55 every morning to wake up your body, and the stretch on page 60 every night to help open the bowels the following morning. Take time each day to practise the guided visualization. In all, aim to work up to at least 30 minutes BRS a day, finding a pattern that suits you, and don't forget that you can combine it with any of the exercises in Chapter 6 too.

Opening up your skin

You can add to all this great work with a daily skin scrub in the bath or shower. Buy a loofah or natural-bristle skin brush and give your skin a gentle scrub, with a natural bath or shower gel, each morning. Exfoliating the dead skin cells and opening up your skin allows it to breathe and act as an organ of elimination. Don't overdo the scrubbing and end up with raw, red skin, and stay away from tender areas, but do try to finish with the skin slightly red and tingling.

THE FOUR-WEEK DETOX MENU PLAN

Use the menu plans from the weekend and week detoxes for your first week; here are the menu plans for weeks two to four. Begin each day with a detox juice or smoothie (see pp.66–9) and end each day with a detox tea (see pp.76–7). Rules on snacks and desserts apply as they did for the shorter detox plans: eat seeds, nuts and crudités for snacks, and a piece of fruit half an hour after your main dinner course for dessert. Feel free to juggle the recipes according to your preference, but try to make sure that you eat a wide variety – try not to stick to just your favourites.

WEEK TWO

DAY	BREAKFAST	LUNCH	DINNER
Monday	Berry fruit salad (p.64)	Persian rice with tomato saffron sauce (p.70)	Roast salmon and beetroot (beet) salad (p.74)
Tuesday	Max's muesli (p.65)	Refreshing watermelon salad (p.71)	Chicken Waldorf salad (p.73)
Wednesday	Green fruit salad (p.64)	Sardines with pomegranate salsa (p.71)	Griddled tuna with Italian five-bean salad (p.73)
Thursday	Egg on toast (p.65)	Soup au pistou (p.72)	Three-bean chilli with avocado salsa (p.75)
Friday	Berry fruit salad (p.64)	Refreshing watermelon salad (p.71)	Really red risotto (p.74)
Saturday	Green fruit salad (p.64)	Ginger chicken skewers with quinoa tabbouleh (p.72)	Roast salmon and beetroot (beet) salad (p.74)
Sunday	Max's muesli (p.65)	Persian rice with tomato saffron sauce (p.70)	Chicken Waldorf salad (p.73)

WEEK THREE

DAY	BREAKFAST	LUNCH	DINNER
Monday	Berry fruit salad (p.64)	Refreshing watermelon salad (p.71)	Griddled tuna with Italian five-bean salad (p.73)
Tuesday	Green fruit salad (p.64)	Ginger chicken skewers with quinoa tabbouleh (p.72)	Really red risotto (p.74)
Wednesday	Egg on toast (p.65)	Soup au pistou (p.72)	Roast salmon and beetroot (beet) salad (p.74)
Thursday	Berry fruit salad (p.64)	Garlic grilled (broiled) sardines with pomegranate salsa (p.71)	Three-bean chilli with avocado salsa (p.75)
Friday	Green fruit salad (p.64)	Soup au pistou (p.72)	Griddle tuna with Italian five-bean salad (p.73)
Saturday	Max's muesli (p.65)	Persian rice with tomato saffron sauce (p.70)	Chicken Waldorf salad (p.73)
Sunday	Berry fruit salad (p.64)	Refreshing watermelon salad (p.71)	Really red risotto (p.74)

WEEK FOUR

DAY	BREAKFAST	LUNCH	DINNER
Monday	Green fruit salad (p.64)	Garlic grilled (broiled) sardines with pomegranate salsa (p.71)	Three-bean chilli with avocado salsa (p.75)
Tuesday	Egg on toast (p.65)	Persian rice with tomato saffron sauce (p.70)	Roast salmon and beetroot (beet) salad (p.74)
Wednesday	Berry fruit salad (p.64)	Ginger chicken skewers with quinoa tabbouleh (p.72)	Griddled tuna with Italian five-bean salad (p.73)
Thursday	Green fruit salad (p.64)	Soup au pistou (p.72)	Chicken Waldorf salad (p.73)
Friday	Berry fruit salad (p.64)	Refreshing watermelon salad (p.71)	Three-bean chilli with avocado salsa (p.75)
Saturday	Max's muesli (p.65)	Garlic grilled (broiled) sardines with pomegranate salsa (p.71)	Really red risotto (p.74)
Sunday	Green fruit salad (p.64)	Persian rice with tomato saffron sauce (p.70)	Griddled tuna with Italian five- bean salad (p.73)

DETOX BREAKFASTS

Berry fruit salad

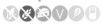

SERVES 1
PREPARATION TIME 5 MINUTES

5 blueberries

5 blackberries

5 raspberries

5 strawberries

5 cherries, stoned

1 green apple

1 pear

1 heaped tsp chopped, raw nuts (use a mixture of almonds, Brazils and hazelnuts)

2 tbsp freshly squeezed orange juice (optional)

1   Wash all the fruit, halve the strawberries and cherries and core and slice the apple and pear.

2   Sprinkle the fruit with the nuts. If you are using it, add the orange juice to flavour.

Green fruit salad

SERVES 1
PREPARATION TIME 5 MINUTES

1 kiwi

1 apple

1 pear

10 green grapes

½ grapefruit

1 tsp chopped, raw seeds (use sunflower seeds, pumpkin seeds and pine nuts)

2 tbsp freshly squeezed orange juice (optional)

1   Wash all the fruit and finely slice the kiwi and core and slice the apple and pear; halve the grapes and segment the grapefruit.

2   Place all the fruit in a bowl and sprinkle with the seeds.

3   If you are using it, add the orange juice.

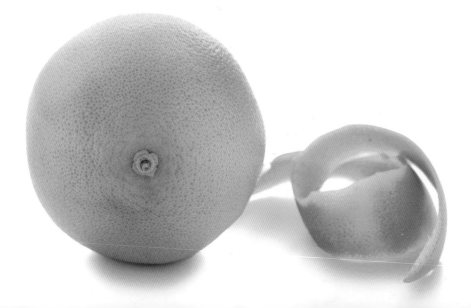

Egg on toast

SERVES 1
PREPARATION TIME 5 MINUTES
COOKING TIME 5 MINUTES

1 or 2 slices wheat-free, wholemeal, yeast-free bread
1 or 2 organic free-range eggs
1 tsp apple cider vinegar
1 tbsp extra virgin olive oil
1 medium clove garlic
1 large tomato, sliced
2 leaves cos (romaine) lettuce

1 Pour some water into a shallow pan (make sure there is enough water to cover the eggs), add the cider vinegar and bring to a light boil.

2 Crack open and gently drop the eggs into the water, one at a time if you are using two. With a spoon, gently nudge the egg whites closer to their yolks. This will help the egg whites hold together. Turn off the heat. Cover.

3 Let the eggs sit in the water for 3 minutes, until the egg whites are cooked. In the meantime, toast the bread.

4 Crush the clove of garlic into the oil, give it a stir and using a pastry brush spread the mixture on the toast.

5 Carefully take the eggs out of the pan using a slotted spoon, place them on the toast and garnish with shredded lettuce and sliced tomato.

Max's muesli

SERVES 2
PREPARATION TIME 10 MINUTES
COOKING TIME 15 MINUTES

1 cup rolled oats
1 heaped tsp pine nuts
½ tsp sesame seeds
4 strawberries
1 tangerine
2 dried apricots, soaked in water overnight
6 fresh cranberries (if available)
1 guava
2 prunes
1 peach
1 plum
Freshly pressed juice of 1 apple

1 Pre-heat the oven to 200°C/fan 180°C/400°F/ gas 6. Spread the rolled oats on a baking tray and place them in the oven, stirring regularly, until they are light golden brown (about 10 minutes).

2 Add the pine nuts and sesame seeds to the tray for the last 4 minutes, mixing them well into the oats to stop them burning.

3 Wash all the fruit and chop it into chunks as necessary. Put it in a bowl and mix it with the baked oats mixture.

4 Add apple juice to taste and allow it to soften the oats before eating.

DETOX JUICES

Hot lemon and ginger

SERVES 1
PREPARATION TIME 5 MINUTES

1 tsp freshly grated root ginger
Juice of 1 whole lemon (pips removed)

1 Add the ginger to a cup of hot water and allow it to soak for 5 minutes.

2 Pour in all the lemon juice, stir and serve.

Green and clean

SERVES 1
PREPARATION TIME 5 MINUTES

Handful spinach
Handful parsley
2 stalks celery
3 carrots

Juice all the ingredients together and pour into your glass.

NOTE: This is one of the harsher-tasting juices – but it is packed with plenty of alkalizing nutrients to help restore the acid–alkaline balance necessary for a healthy body (see pp.86–7), so drink it as often as you can during your detox.

Green power

SERVES 1
PREPARATION TIME 5 MINUTES

½ head of cos (romaine) lettuce

1 green or red apple

1 small cucumber

3 stalks celery

3 small spinach leaves

Small handful parsley

½ large carrot or 1 small carrot (optional)

½ clove garlic (optional)

1 Juice the lettuce first, then the apples (if you are using the garlic, add this now too).

2 Slowly add the rest of the ingredients to the juicer and juice them gently to make sure you extract all of the juice. Pour into a glass and serve.

Super-cleanse

SERVES 1
PREPARATION TIME 5 MINUTES

2 carrots

½ cucumber

1 fresh beetroot (beet)

Small (2.5cm/1in) stick ginger (optional)

1 clove garlic, crushed and left to stand for 5 minutes before juicing (optional)

1 Wash the vegetables carefully.

2 Juice the carrots, cucumber and beetroot (beet).

3 Add the ginger and garlic if you are using them, stir and then pour into your glass.

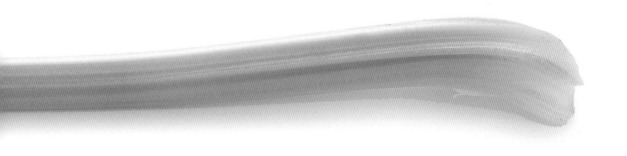

DETOX SMOOTHIES

Cleansing cocktail

SERVES 1
PREPARATION TIME 2 MINUTES

100% cranberry juice (no added sugar), diluted one
part cranberry to three parts water

2 tsp psyllium husks

Pour the cranberry and water mixture into a
large glass and tip in the psyllium husks. Stir
well and drink quickly.

Pink mango smoothie

SERVES 1
PREPARATION TIME 5 MINUTES

1 ripe mango, pitted
1 pink grapefruit

1 Purée the mango.

2 Juice the grapefruit, removing the pith.

3 Mix the two together well and pour into a glass.
When you drink, sip the mixture, so that you
mix it with your saliva (the enzymes in the
mango help to cleanse the tongue, which may
become coated during the detox).

Pure and simple

SERVES 1
PREPARATION TIME 2 MINUTES
COOKING TIME 5 MINUTES

2 apples
2.5cm/1in fresh ginger
½ a ripe banana, puréed
½ a freshly squeezed lemon
Dash freshly squeezed orange juice

1 Juice the apples and ginger.

2 Mix well with the puréed banana and add the
lemon and orange juice and serve.

Pineapple and pear perfection

SERVES 1
PREPARATION TIME 5 MINUTES

1 cup fresh, ripe pineapple chunks
1 ripe pear
6 crushed blueberries

1 Purée the pineapple and pear together.

2 Crush the blueberries and stir into the pineapple
mixture. Pour into a glass. As you drink, "chew"
the smoothie so that the enzymes in the
pineapple help to cleanse your tongue.

PANG: Pineapple, apple and ginger

SERVES 1
PREPARATION TIME 5 MINUTES

1cm/½in fresh ginger root
1 apple
⅛ large pineapple

1 Peel the ginger and pineapple. Wash the apple well. Slice the apple and pineapple.

2 Juice the ginger first, then the fruit. Stir in the froth and drink immediately.

PAF: Plums, apple, figs

SERVES 1
PREPARATION TIME 5 MINUTES

2 or 3 ripe figs
2 ripe plums, washed and stoned
1 apple, washed and seeded

1 Scoop out the flesh of the figs and purée them in a food processor.

2 Juice the plums and apple.

3 Pour the juice over the figs and stir well. Pour into a glass and serve.

CCC: Celery, cabbage, carrots

SERVES 1
PREPARATION TIME 5 MINUTES

4 sticks celery
¼ cabbage
2 carrots

1 Wash all the vegetables thoroughly and then chop them into small pieces.

2 Juice them all together, stir, pour into a glass, and drink immediately.

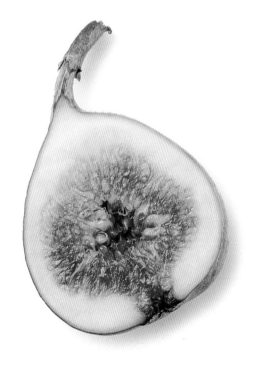

DETOX LUNCHES

Persian rice with tomato saffron sauce

SERVES 2
PREPARATION TIME 30 MINUTES
COOKING TIME 1 HOUR

140g/5oz/⅔ cup brown rice, rinsed

4 tbsp green lentils, rinsed

2 bay leaves

1 litre/35 fl oz/4½ cups water

1 medium onion, peeled and finely sliced

1 small onion, peeled and chopped

2 tbsp extra virgin olive oil

450g/1lb ripe tomatoes

2 tbsp pine nuts, lightly toasted

2 tbsp unsalted pistachio nuts, lightly toasted

20 gratings nutmeg

2 tbsp plus 2 tsp lemon juice

2 pinches saffron threads

Small bunch coriander (cilantro), to serve

1   Put the rice, lentils, bay leaves and 900ml/
30 fl oz/3¾ cups of water in a saucepan over a
medium heat. Bring to the boil, then reduce the
heat slightly, cover and simmer for 40 minutes,
until the rice is tender.

2   Meanwhile, put the sliced onion, half the olive oil
and 150ml/5 fl oz/¾ cup water in a 20cm/8in frying
pan (skillet) over a medium to low heat and cook
gently for 30 minutes, stirring occasionally, until the
onions are soft and sweet. Increase the heat to
high and boil off any excess water, then cook the
onions for 7–8 minutes until brown and
caramelized. Watch them carefully and stir
frequently to prevent them burning.

3   While the onion and rice are cooking, skin the
tomatoes. Cut a cross in the top of each tomato
and put them in a large heatproof bowl. Pour over
enough boiling water to cover and leave for 10
seconds. Remove the tomatoes from the water

using a slotted spoon, and peel off the skin
when they are cool enough to handle. Discard
the seeds and roughly chop the tomato flesh.

4   Drain the rice and remove the bay leaves. Stir in
the pine nuts, pistachios, caramelized onions,
nutmeg and 2 tbsp lemon juice. Keep warm in a
very low oven until the tomato sauce is ready.

5   Put the chopped onion and remaining olive oil in
a medium saucepan over a low heat and cook
for 10 minutes, until softened. Add the saffron
and cook for 2 minutes. Add the tomatoes, raise
the heat to medium and cook for 5 minutes,
until the tomatoes have softened slightly but
have not collapsed. Stir in 2 tsp lemon juice.

6   Divide the rice between two plates and spoon
over the tomato sauce. Scatter over the
coriander (cilantro) before serving.

Refreshing watermelon salad

SERVES 2
PREPARATION TIME 25 MINUTES

360g/13oz/3 cups cubed watermelon

2 small pink grapefruits, skin and pith removed and segmented

¼ medium cucumber (110g/4oz), halved and sliced

125g/4½oz firm rindless goat's cheese, broken into 1cm/½in cubes

Small bunch mint, chopped but reserve a few leaves for garnish

1 tbsp extra virgin olive oil

1 tsp lemon juice

1 Put the watermelon, grapefruit, cucumber and goat's cheese into a large bowl.

2 Whisk the mint, olive oil and lemon juice together in a small bowl and pour over the salad ingredients. Gently toss the salad in the dressing and scatter over the reserved mint leaves before serving.

Garlic grilled (broiled) sardines with pomegranate salsa

SERVES 2
PREPARATION TIME 20 MINUTES
COOKING TIME 8 MINUTES

½ pomegranate, seeds removed

Small bunch coriander (cilantro), chopped

Very small bunch flat leaf parsley, chopped

3 salad onions, trimmed and finely sliced

½ red chilli, diced (for medium heat)

2 tbsp lemon juice

2 medium cloves garlic, peeled and crushed

2 tsp extra virgin olive oil

4 x 110g/4oz sardines, de-scaled and gutted

2 large handfuls rocket (40g/1½oz)

2 lemon quarters, to serve

1 Put the pomegranate seeds, coriander (cilantro), parsley, onions and chilli in a small bowl. Stir in the lemon juice.

2 Preheat the grill (broiler) to high. Mix together the garlic and olive oil and brush over the outside of the sardines. Grill (broil) the sardines for 3–4 minutes on each side, until cooked through.

3 Divide the rocket between two plates and lay the sardines on top. Spoon over the salsa and serve with the lemon quarters.

Soup au pistou

SERVES 2
PREPARATION TIME 15 MINUTES (PLUS OVERNIGHT SOAKING)
COOKING TIME 2 HOURS 5 MINUTES (INCLUDES 1 HOUR 40 MINUTES COOKING TIME FOR BEANS)

4 tbsp haricot beans
1 small onion, peeled and finely chopped
1 small carrot, peeled and finely chopped
1 large stick celery, finely chopped
1 medium courgette (zucchini), finely chopped
1 tbsp plus 2 tsp extra virgin olive oil
1 medium clove garlic, peeled and crushed
600ml/20 fl oz/2½ cups vegetable stock
2 sprigs thyme
1 medium tomato, deseeded and finely chopped
4 tsp lemon juice
Small bunch basil, leaves roughly torn
2 tsp pine nuts, lightly toasted (optional)

1 Soak the beans overnight and cook according to the recipe on p.75 (step 2).

2 Put the onion, carrot, celery, courgette (zucchini) and 1 tbsp olive oil in a large pan over a low heat and cook for 10 minutes, until the vegetables start to soften. Add the garlic and cook for 1 minute.

3 Add the stock, thyme and drained beans. Increase the heat to medium and simmer for 10 minutes. Add the tomato and cook for a further 5 minutes. Stir in the lemon juice. Remove the thyme sprigs.

4 Put the basil leaves in a small bowl and mix in the remaining olive oil with the pine nuts (optional). Ladle the soup into two large bowls and spoon over the basil mixture to serve.

Ginger chicken skewers with quinoa tabbouleh

SERVES 2
PREPARATION TIME 20 MINUTES (PLUS 15–30 MINUTES MARINATING)
COOKING TIME 25 MINUTES

2 x 110g/4oz skinless organic chicken breasts, cut into 1cm/½in cubes
4 tbsp plus 2 tsp extra virgin olive oil
4 tbsp plus 2 tsp lemon juice
½ medium clove garlic, peeled and crushed
1 tsp fresh ginger, grated
½ tsp ground ginger
85g/3oz/⅓ cup quinoa, rinsed
150ml/5 fl oz/⅔ cup water
Large bunch flat leaf parsley, chopped
Large bunch coriander (cilantro), chopped
Large bunch mint, chopped
6 salad onions, trimmed and finely sliced
2 lemon quarters, to serve

1 Soak four wooden skewers in water for 10 minutes. Put the chicken, 2 tsp olive oil, 2 tsp lemon juice, the garlic and both gingers in a small bowl and stir to coat the chicken in the marinade. Leave to stand for 15–30 minutes.

2 Cook the quinoa (see packet instructions). Spread out on a plate and cool for 10 minutes. Put the chopped herbs, onions and cooled quinoa in a bowl and stir in 4 tbsp olive oil and 4 tbsp lemon juice.

3 Preheat the grill (broiler) to high. Skewer the chicken and grill (broil) for 3–4 minutes on each side, until cooked through and golden. Divide the tabbouleh between two plates and top with two chicken skewers. Serve with the lemon.

DETOX DINNERS

Chicken Waldorf salad

SERVES 2
PREPARATION TIME 15 MINUTES
COOKING TIME 20 MINUTES

2 x 110g/4oz skinless, boneless organic chicken breasts
1 fat clove garlic, peeled and sliced
Small bunch tarragon
600ml/20 fl oz/2½ cups water
3 medium sticks celery, thinly sliced
1 medium green apple, cored and cut into thin slices
1 medium bunch seedless green grapes (250g/9oz), halved
4 tbsp live goat's yogurt
2 tsp lemon juice

1 Put the chicken breasts in a medium saucepan with the garlic and half the tarragon. Add the water and place over a medium heat. Simmer for 20 minutes, turning the chicken over halfway through. Put the chicken on a plate and allow to cool for 10 minutes.

2 Slice the chicken thinly and put in a large bowl with the celery, apple and grapes.

3 Chop the remaining tarragon leaves and whisk with the yogurt and lemon juice in a small bowl. Spoon over the salad and toss gently before serving.

Griddled tuna with Italian five-bean salad

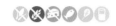

SERVES 2
PREPARATION TIME 15 MINUTES (PLUS OVERNIGHT SOAKING)
COOKING TIME 2 HOURS (INCLUDES 1 HOUR 30 MINUTES SIMMERING TIME FOR BEANS)

2 tbsp each dried kidney beans, dried flageolet beans, dried canellini beans, dried chickpeas (garbanzos)
Large handful (85g/3oz) green beans
½ medium red onion, peeled and finely chopped
1 fat clove garlic, crushed
3 tbsp extra virgin olive oil
2 tbsp fresh lemon juice
2 x 150g/5oz line-caught yellow fin tuna steaks, cut 5cm/2in thick
Small bunch flat leaf parsley, roughly chopped
2 lemon quarters, to serve

1 Soak the dried beans overnight and cook according to the recipe on page 75 (step 2). Cut the green beans into 2.5cm/1in lengths and add for the final 2–3 minutes cooking time. Drain all the beans and rinse with cold water.

2 Put the beans in a bowl and stir in the onion, garlic, 2 tbsp olive oil and 1 tbsp lemon juice. Stand for 15 minutes.

3 Preheat a griddle pan. Griddle the tuna for 2 minutes (medium-rare) on each side.

4 Add the remaining 1 tbsp each of lemon juice and olive oil and the parsley to the beans and stir well. Spoon onto two plates; top with the tuna. Serve with the lemon quarters.

Really red risotto

SERVES 2
PREPARATION TIME 20 MINUTES
COOKING TIME 40 MINUTES

1 medium red onion, peeled and finely chopped
1 tbsp extra virgin olive oil
1 fat clove garlic, peeled and crushed
150g/5½oz/¾ cup Camargue red rice, rinsed
450ml/15 fl oz/1⅞ cups vegetable stock
2 sprigs thyme, leaves chopped
1 medium red (bell) pepper (110g/4oz), halved and seeds removed
10 baby plum tomatoes (110g/4oz), quartered
1 tbsp lemon juice
Small bunch parsley, chopped

1 Put the onion and olive oil in a medium saucepan over a low heat and cook gently for 7 minutes. Add the garlic and rice and cook for a further 2 minutes. Add the stock and thyme, increase the heat to medium and simmer for 25 minutes.

2 Meanwhile, preheat the grill (broiler) to high and grill (broil) the skin side of the pepper for 3–4 minutes until blistering. Put in a large bowl and cover with a plate and leave for 5–6 minutes, then peel the skin off the pepper. Cut the flesh into thin slices.

3 Add the pepper to the rice and cook for a further 8 minutes, until the rice is tender. Add the tomatoes and cook for 2 minutes. Stir in the lemon juice and parsley just before serving.

Roast salmon and beetroot (beet) salad

SERVES 2
PREPARATION TIME 10 MINUTES
COOKING TIME 1 HOUR 10 MINUTES

4 small beetroot (beet), unpeeled (4 x 70g/2½oz)
1 medium red onion, unpeeled
2 x 110g/4oz organic salmon fillets
2 tbsp plus 2 tsp extra virgin olive oil
2 large handfuls watercress
2 tsp cider vinegar

1 Preheat the oven to 200°C/fan 180°C/400°F/gas 6. Put the beetroot (beet) on a flat baking sheet and roast in the top of the oven for 30 minutes. Add the onion and roast for a further 30 minutes, until tender. Remove from the oven and allow to cool slightly.

2 Brush the salmon with 2 tsp of the olive oil, put on a flat baking sheet and roast in the same oven for 10–12 minutes, until the salmon is cooked and just starting to flake.

3 Meanwhile, peel the cooked onion and beetroot (beet) with a sharp knife (wear rubber gloves to prevent the beetroot staining your hands) and cut each into eight pieces.

4 Put the watercress, warm onion, and beetroot (beet) in a large bowl. Whisk the vinegar and remaining olive oil together in a small bowl, pour over the salad and toss well. Divide between two plates and flake the salmon over the top.

Three-bean chilli with avocado salsa

SERVES 2
PREPARATION TIME 25 MINUTES (PLUS OVERNIGHT SOAKING)
COOKING TIME 1 HOUR

3 tbsp pinto beans

3 tbsp black beans

3 tbsp black-eye peas

½ small onion, peeled and finely chopped

1 large stick celery, finely chopped

1 tbsp extra virgin olive oil

1 tsp ground cumin

¼ tsp paprika

1 fat clove garlic, crushed

½ fresh red chilli, deseeded and finely chopped

450ml/15 fl oz/1⅞ cups vegetable stock

1 bay leaf

110g/4oz/¾ cup brown rice

½ medium avocado, peeled, stoned and cut into small cubes

4 salad onions, trimmed and finely sliced

Small bunch coriander (cilantro), chopped

1 tbsp lime juice

2 lime quarters, to serve

1 Put the dried beans into a large bowl and cover with plenty of cold water. Leave to soak for 12 hours, or overnight. They should roughly double in volume.

2 Drain the beans and rinse well, then put them in a large saucepan. Cover with fresh cold water. Put over a high heat and bring to the boil. Boil rapidly for 10 minutes.

3 Put the onion, celery and olive oil in a large saucepan and cook over a medium heat for 5 minutes. Add the cumin and paprika and cook for 2 minutes, then add the garlic and chilli and cook for 1 minute.

4 Drain the beans and rinse them again, then add to the onion mixture. Pour over the vegetable stock and add the bay leaf. Place over a medium heat and bring up to a simmer. Cook uncovered for 1 hour, until the beans have softened. Add a little extra stock if the beans become dry. By the end of cooking there should be 2–3 tbsp of liquid left.

5 Cook the brown rice according to the packet instructions. Drain and keep warm.

6 Put the avocado, salad onions, coriander (cilantro) and lime juice in a small bowl and mix together.

7 Divide the rice between two plates or bowls and spoon over the bean chilli. Top with the avocado salsa and serve with the lime quarters.

NOTE: This makes a fairly mild chilli. To increase the heat, use chilli powder instead of paprika and increase the amount of fresh red chilli to suit your own taste.

DETOX TEAS

As this is a detox, it wouldn't be appropriate to undo all your good work with a host of sweet desserts. So, in this chapter we have swapped the dessert recipes for some cleansing herbal teas.

Detox me tea

SERVES 1
PREPARATION TIME 5 MINUTES
COOKING TIME 20 MINUTES

1 part roasted dandelion root (*Taraxacum officinale*)
1 part burdock root (*Arctium lappa*)
¼ part ginger root (*Zingiber officinale*)
¼ part clove bud (*Syzgium aromaticum*)
1 part horsetail herb (*Equisetum arvense*)
¼ part dried orange peel
2 pieces of cinnamon bark (*Cinnamomum cassia*)

1 Pour 570 ml/20 fl oz/3 cups distilled or purified water into a stainless steel pot.

2 Add 2 tbsp of the tea herbs to the water, cover the pot and let the mixture soak overnight. In the morning bring the mixture to the boil and then reduce the heat and simmer gently for 20 minutes.

3 Using a strainer, pour the tea into a mug, and drink while hot.

4 Put the strained, wet herbs back into the pot and keep them in the refrigerator. You may reuse the herbs for up to 3 days.

Pure foods detox tea

SERVES 1
PREPARATION TIME 2 MINUTES
COOKING TIME 5 MINUTES

1 part aniseed seed (*Pimpinella anisum*)
1 part fennel seed (*Foeniculum officinale*)
1 part cardamom seed (*Elettaria cardamomum*)
1 part coriander seed (*Coriandrum sativum*)
1 part licorice root, finely chopped (*Glycyrrhiza glabra*)
1 part celery seed (*Apium graveolens*)

1 Combine the dried herbs in a small bowl.

2 Place 1 tsp of the mixture in a big mug of hot water. Allow it to soak for 5 minutes and then strain and drink.

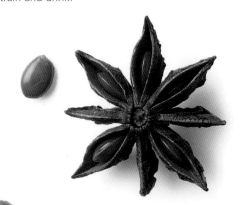

Tangy tea

SERVES 1
PREPARATION TIME 2 MINUTES

1 tbsp real, organic maple syrup
Juice of ½ a lemon
Tiny pinch of cayenne pepper to taste (you will need hardly any – be careful, it is very strong and hot!)

Mix the ingredients together in a mug, pour over hot water, stir and drink.

African delight

SERVES 1
PREPARATION TIME 2 MINUTES
COOKING TIME 5 MINUTES

1 tea bag organic rooibos tea
Dash fresh orange juice

Place the teabag in a big mug of boiling water. Allow it to soak for 5 minutes, add the fresh orange juice to taste, and serve.

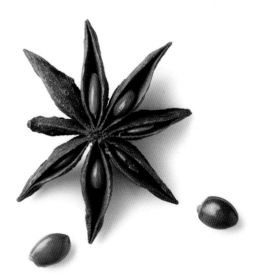

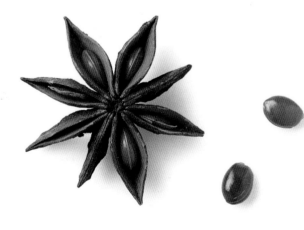

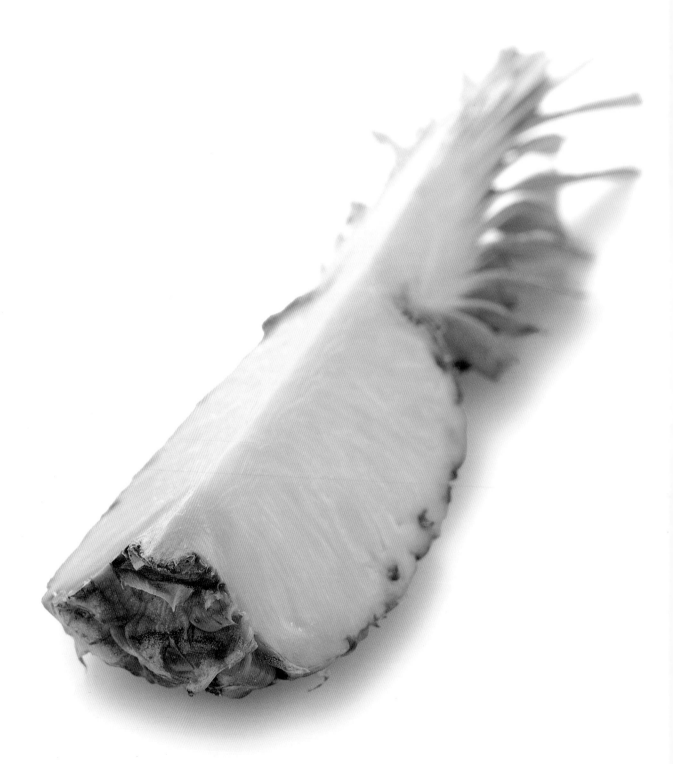

the digestion tune-up plans

make use of the amazing power of pure foods to heal your digestive tract

DO YOU NEED TO HEAL YOUR DIGESTION?

ARE YOU:

Often bloated and embarrassingly flatulent?

Suffering from constipation or diarrhea?

Allergic or sensitive to certain foods?

Worried about aches and pains in your stomach?

Up at night with heartburn?

Scared to eat lunch as you feel so tired and sluggish afterward?

Think you've taken too many antibiotics in the past?

Concerned about a family history of bowel cancer?

Just not sure what to eat any more as it seems as though most foods cause you discomfort?

If you answered yes to any of these questions, this section will help you understand your digestive problem and may help you to find a permanent solution. In naturopathic terms, your digestion is paramount to your overall health.

HOW DIGESTION WORKS

Digestion is one of our most complicated body systems. It begins
with the eyes, nose and mouth, and includes the esophagus,
stomach, small and large intestines, pancreas, liver and gall
bladder. Pure foods can help to keep them all working optimally.

A beginner's guide to digestion

SIGHT AND SMELL The sight and smell of food stimulate your digestive
tract and get the digestive juices flowing. This is why it is so important to look
at your food before eating it, so that the digestive process can begin properly.

MOUTH Saliva contains an enzyme that starts to break down carbohydrates
in the mouth. If you have ever chewed a piece of bread for a while you will
have noticed that it gets quite sweet as the carbohydrates break down into
simpler sugars. I am sure that proper mastication (chewing) would sort out a lot
of common digestive problems, so take time to chew. Incidentally, your tongue
is a wonderful barometer of your digestive health. The tongue in a healthy
body appears soft, pink and wet. But if your tongue is dry, yellowed and
cracked, you could well be in urgent need of a digestive overhaul.

ESOPHAGUS When you swallow and your food leaves your mouth, it enters
the esophagus. This long pipe connects your mouth to your stomach and is
lined with a delicate mucous membrane that helps the food to slide down. If
your stomach rejects the food, it travels back up as vomit – a mixture of food,
caustic stomach acids and digestive enzymes that can damage the esophagus
lining. Acid reflux (heartburn), where stomach acids travel up the esophagus,
also damages the delicate lining. Don't ignore reflux of any sort, as it can lead
to ulceration and even cancer.

"Without a properly functioning digestive system, you cannot be healthy. Fact."

STOMACH I always ask clients to tell me where they think their stomachs are. Near the belly button? No – your stomach is surprisingly high up under the ribcage. It is a type of living cement mixer: the stomach muscles churn your food, mixing it with hydrochloric acid, protective mucus, and protein-digesting enzymes, as well as special hormones that control the whole show. This process starts the breakdown of foods into smaller component parts, which the intestines can then absorb into your blood stream.

SMALL INTESTINE Small is a silly name for the longest part of your bowel – it is 6m (18ft) long! This, the most exciting part of the digestive system, is where all the digestive action takes place, with proteins, carbohydrates and fats being broken down into tiny component parts. The absorption of these digested nutrients into the blood stream begins in the small intestine.

LARGE INTESTINE The large intestine plays no actual role in digestion itself, but it still holds an important role in the absorption of water and mineral salts from the stool as it passes through. It also helps to periodically remove bacteria from the bowel during each bowel motion and temporarily stores feces and undigested material before we excrete it. To be frank, this is the smelly, nasty section of the bowel and full of bacteria – and that is just in healthy people!

LIVER AND GALL BLADDER The liver is the primary organ of digestion as it helps the body to digest and store nutrients. For example, the liver stores vitamins (except vitamin C), iron and several other minerals until the body requires them, as well as storing glucose (as glycogen), which the body needs for energy. It also forms bile salts, which are then stored in the gall bladder until we need them to help with the digestion of fats.

PANCREAS The pancreas supports digestion by producing digestive enzymes that break down our food and an alkaline liquid to reduce the acidity of the food after it leaves the stomach and enters the small intestine. It also produces hormones, such as insulin, that help with the metabolism of carbohydrate.

If there is a problem with any of these elements of digestion, or with any part of the process of elimination (see Detox), we may suffer bloating, wind, bad breath and tiredness – among other things. But why might problems occur?

What can affect our digestion?

STRESS AND TENSION These have a huge impact on digestive health. When we feel stressed, the body enters the fight-or-flight mode. This takes blood and circulation away from the digestive tract and into the muscles and brain so that the arms can fight, the legs can run and the head think. When the digestive tract has a drastically reduced blood supply, it produces fewer digestive enzymes. The result is that food is not properly broken down and digested in the stomach and small intestine, so that when it eventually enters the large intestine it sits there rotting and fermenting, and not being digested, causing bloating, discomfort and irritation to the lining of the bowels. Poor liver function (including ineffective removal of toxins by the liver) and dehydration, both of which can greatly increase the time it takes to move food and stool through the small and large intestines, just add to the problem. The longer wastes sit in the large intestine, the greater the chance that you will reabsorb from the stool the very toxins you are trying to eliminate.

GOOD AND BAD BACTERIA Probiotics – so-called friendly bacteria, or good flora – are hugely important in digestive health. We have more than 100 trillion bacteria (comprising 400 different bacterial species) in the digestive tract. These bacteria enhance the breakdown and absorption of vitamins and proteins and produce substances that help to reduce cholesterol and regulate blood sugars. They also keep in check the unfriendly bacteria (bad flora), which thrive on sugar, alcohol and refined foods, and can cause bloating and flatulence and even conditions such as irritable bowel syndrome. Good flora are damaged by such things as antibiotics, the contraceptive pill, and a poor

"Digestion begins with savouring your food before you eat it."

diet. When this happens we stop absorbing nutrients properly and bad bacteria can flourish, leading to problems such irritable bowel syndrome (see below).

Poor digestion, poor you!

Poor digestion, and an increase in negative bacteria and fungi in the digestive tract, lead to food rotting and fermenting in the intestines. Fermentation creates chemical by-products that irritate the linings of the intestines, which may in the long-term lead to irritable bowel syndrome (IBS). If the lining of the bowel becomes very damaged, we may develop a "leaking gut", in which the damaged bowel lining allows partially digested food through directly into the blood stream. The immune system takes a dim view of this invasion, initiating an immune response to the food particles. Your immunity sees the leaked food as an antigen (an unwanted invader), and you may ultimately develop an allergy to it. This means that each time you eat this particular food, your immune system goes on full alert to protect you and you feel tired because of the huge amount of energy directed into defending you. The weaker and more tired you are, the more chance the bad flora have to thrive – and so it goes on. (Of course, leaky gut is not the only cause of food allergens. Many of us suffer the symptoms of sensitivity: bloating, tiredness, pain, and perhaps even skin complaints such as acne or eczema, for which there are various causes, including genetic disposition and simple overexposure to certain foods. Constant exposure to the same proteins and sugars in a limited range of foods can create a sensitivity. Remember: "familiarity breeds contempt".)

Switching to pure foods

So, how can eating pure foods help your digestive crisis? The answer is simple. Clean, pure, low-allergy foods and drinks reduce the strain on the digestive tract because they come complete with the natural enzymes, vitamins and minerals that aid digestion. Their nutrients are in as natural a state as possible, which makes them easier for the body to absorb, thus reducing the strain on the digestive system; and they do not come with any of the nasty chemicals or preservatives that hamper the process of digestion. All this, in turn, enables the good flora to flourish, and all parts of the digestive system to work at their optimum levels. Pure foods are just plain easier to digest.

How the digestion plans work

Over the following pages are the three digestion tune-up plans, one lasting a weekend (see pp.90–93), one a week (pp.96–8) and one a month (pp.99–101).

WHICH PLAN SHOULD I USE – WEEKEND, WEEK OR MONTH?
The weekend plan is ideal for anyone who has suffered a short period of constipation, diarrhea, or other digestive problem. If you have been on antibiotics for a long time or have suffered a prolonged period of bloating, flatulence or heartburn – common symptoms of a digestive problem – but are otherwise fit and healthy, aim for one of the longer plans.

HOW ARE THE PLANS LAID OUT?
The first step in each plan prepares you to get the most out of the plan; the second guides you specifically through the foods you should eat while you are on the plan, and refers to the recipes on pages 102–115; and the third offers breathing, relaxing and stretching advice to complement your tune-up.

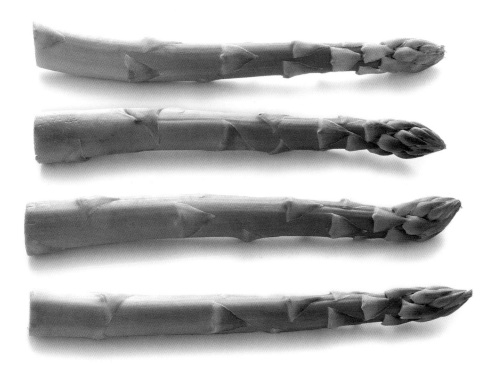

INTRODUCING THE DIGESTION TUNE-UP PLANS

As a naturopath I don't think you can ever do enough to ensure that your stomach and intestines are in fabulous health. In this section I will introduce you to the digestion plans and highlight what benefits you can expect to see as a result of following them.

The benefits of the plans

First and foremost the digestion plans will enable your body to correctly absorb vitamins and minerals from your foods. This alone will bring visible benefits – you will be less bloated, your skin will develop a healthy glow, and you will feel buoyed up with energy. The extra fruit and vegetables in your diet will mean more regular bowel motions. Most impressive of all will be the invisible changes – a gradual reduction in the irritation to the lining of the bowels and so increased resistance to all the health problems it brings (see p.84).

General rules for the plans

HAVE A HEALTHY BREAKFAST During the night your body is busy cleaning and repairing damage to the digestive tract, and breakfast should complement this process. A good healthy breakfast of pure, non-allergenic foods helps the body to start the day in digestive bliss and will give you lots of energy.

PRACTISE FOOD COMBINING IN THE EVENINGS Separating your proteins (meat, fish, chicken, beans) and carbohydrates (bread, pasta, potatoes) at dinner eases the load on your digestive system (see pp.125–6). The stomach produces acids to break down proteins, and alkaline to enable the digestion of carbohydrates. Acid and alkaline neutralize each other in a weakened digestive tract, and this can extend the time it takes to break down food. If your digestive tract is still busy long after dinner, you will find it harder to sleep.

EAT BEFORE 8PM Bed is for sleeping and resting, not digesting. The body does a lot of repair work to the digestive tract at night and this process is retarded if you go to bed with a full stomach.

AVOID SUGAR Glucose and sucrose (table sugar) are of very little use to your body – they promote the growth of the negative bacteria and fungi in the gut. We get all the sugars we need from wholegrains and fruit. However, even fruit sugar (fructose) can create or exacerbate bloating and indigestion, so eat fruit away from your main meals – the negative effect that fruit sugars might have is much weaker when the stomach is empty of other food.

AVOID THE ALLERGENS The protein casein and the sugar lactose in cow's dairy, and the wheat protein gluten (among other constituents of wheat) can cause abdominal bloating, wind, cramping in the lower intestines, bad breath, eczema and lethargy. Drink sheep's, goat's, rice or soya (soy) milk instead of cow's milk; and instead of wheat-based bread, pasta and cereals, eat millet, quinoa, oats, rye and buckwheat, and to a lesser extent kamut and spelt.

AVOID DEADLY NIGHTSHADES These veggies include tomatoes, aubergines (eggplants), capiscums and white potatoes (and tobacco, too!), and contain compounds that can be hard to digest, often leading to bloating. Try to restrict your intake of them as much as possible.

DON'T DRINK WITH MEALS The digestive process involves concentrating digestive juices in the stomach and small intestine. Drinking water with meals dilutes these juices, slowing down digestion. However, this doesn't mean don't drink! You should aim to drink around 2 litres (4 pints) of pure water a day, just avoid drinking at mealtimes.

REMEMBER THAT DIGESTION BEGINS WITH THE EYES, NOSE AND MOUTH Look at your food, smell it, and chew it properly (see p.80).

DON'T EAT STANDING UP OR WALKING   The digestive tract needs a constant and plentiful supply of blood (see p.82). When you stand or walk, blood moves into the muscles of the legs and arms and away from digestion.

Side-effects during the plans

There is always a slight chance of a healing crisis when you clear out your digestive system and your body begins to repair itself. The chances of crises increase the longer the clear-out. You may experience a slight fever and a few aches and pains in the digestive tract. You may find that the increase in vegetable fibre actually exacerbates the amount of wind and bloating you experience for the first few days. Try taking a digestive enzyme complex with each meal (see opposite) and, even if you feel bad at the start of the plan, please persevere – quite soon your bowels will respond positively and normalize. On the longer digestion plans, you will probably experience signs of a general detox, such as runny nose, sore eyes, aches and pains in your joints, headaches, dry skin, minor fever and tiredness (all of these should pass quite quickly). Just rest and drink lots of Max's soothing digestive tea (see p.91).

What's on the menu?

The digestion plan menus are packed full with fibre-rich foods to tackle any signs of constipation or diarrhea. Apricot, carrot, papaya, pineapple, mango, lentils and pumpkin all pack a fibre-fuelled punch. In addition, breakfasts of linseed (flax seed) porridge will help to stimulate the bowel's movements by bulking out the stool, helping it to pass more easily along the intestine. Papaya and pineapple also contain important protein-digesting enzymes (papain and

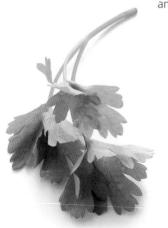
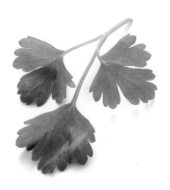
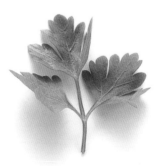

bromelain respectively), which help with the breakdown of food in the gut, maximizing the absorption of nutrients into the rest of the body. We end each day with a cup of my soothing digestive tea (see p.91), which contains the super-digestive herbs peppermint and fennel.

First-aid supplements for the digestion plans

- A digestive enzyme capsule containing protease, cellulase, lipase, lactase, sucrase, amylase and maltase will help to break down proteins, fats, carbohydrates and plant fibre, and so is a really useful aid to prevent bloating after you have eaten. Taken after a meal they ensure trouble-free digestion.
- The herb slippery elm (*Ulmus fulva*) helps to buffer the mucous membranes in the gastrointestinal tract, preventing irritation from foods and assisting the passage of food and stool. Take a good-quality capsule, or a teaspoon of the powder in warm water, before meals.
- Marsh mallow (*Althea officinalis*) is a herbal remedy often used to soothe and heal the lining of the bowels. It is best taken before meals as a herbal liquid (tincture) or as a capsule.
- Probiotics are "friendly" bacteria. The two friendliest bacteria of all (see p.82) are lactobacillus acidophilus and lactobacillus bifidus. These flora help to keep the negative, damaging bacteria under control and so improve digestion. It is very important to buy the best-quality supplement you can afford, containing at least four billion live organisms. These bacteria are sensitive to heat and so the way they are manufactured and stored is very important. Talk to someone at your local health-food store, who should be able to advise you and help you to find a good-quality brand.

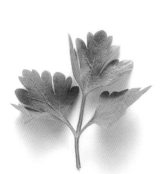 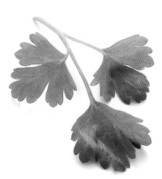 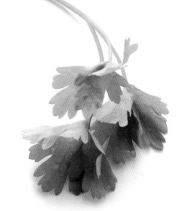

INTRODUCING THE WEEKEND DIGESTION TUNE-UP

This plan covers two days and is ideal if your digestive tract needs a quick fine-tune, if you need to restore digestive health after a particularly heavy eating and drinking session, or if you have suffered a recent viral or bacterial stomach upset.

Why should I do the weekend plan?

This plan is your first step to digestive freedom. I have made a huge effort to make my digestion recipes really gentle on your digestive tract, and in particular as free as possible from allergenic foods (see p.87). Two days should be enough to show you a new way of eating, and a new way of dealing with your digestive problems, whether they are bad breath or constipation, wind or diarrhea. This plan might not be the total digestive cure, but it is a safe and natural beginning to that cure and it will open your eyes to just what is available to you simply by changing what you put into your stomach.

What benefits will I see and feel?

The longer you eat pure foods and give your digestive system a break, the greater the benefits you will experience. However, as I have already said, a weekend is plenty of time to put you on the right track. Your eyes will begin to regain their sparkle, your skin will appear clearer and your hair will shine. Your intestinal bloating will reduce, meaning that your clothes won't feel tight and uncomfortable after a meal or toward the end of the day, and your bowel motions will become calmer and more regular. The need for something sugary at the end of a meal should pass, as your sugar levels stabilize and you feel more contented after eating. You should also feel less tired once you've eaten.

Finishing the digestion plans

First and foremost, do a great thing for your digestion and make Monday the finishing line, and not Sunday – your bowels will appreciate the extra hours of overnight detoxing. Then, don't rush out and eat every type of food that you've missed or dreamed of! Your long-term vitality largely depends upon the health of your digestive tract – so much so that the first naturopaths would begin treating everyone by working on digestion and elimination. After you have completed the weekend plan, by all means reintroduce some of the foods we have removed, but do so with care. If anything makes you feel bloated or flatulent, think about keeping this food out for a little longer. Try to keep going beyond the plan with some of the good principles of diet – munch those fruit and veg, eat plenty of fibre-rich foods and drink lots of water.

After the week or month plans, you will have a completely clean digestive slate (the weekend isn't really long enough to wipe out all the baddies), so use the opportunity to begin a food and drink diary. Be specific about what you ingest – note down *everything* you eat and drink – and in particular try not to forget those snacks that simply slip in while you aren't thinking. Write down how you feel throughout the day, even if it seems unrelated – food sensitivities may cause anything from bloating and flatulence to headaches, feelings of sadness and even (at the extreme) bleeding from the bowel. After a few weeks take your food diary along to a naturopath or nutritionist to review; or simply work out yourself, by a process of elimination, which foods appear to be especially bad for you – and then cut them out of your diet.

MAX'S SOOTHING DIGESTIVE TEA

Peppermint is an age-old stomach settler, while chamomile will calm any stress-related digestive problems and fennel will ease wind or abdominal pain. Drink this tea after your meals as a settling digestive.

To prepare the dried tea, mix together equal parts of the dried, organic herbs peppermint, chamomile and fennel. Add orange peel to taste.

When you are ready to make the tea, place a teaspoon of the dried herb mixture per cup in a tea pot. Allow the tea to steep for five minutes in hot water before drinking.

THE WEEKEND DIGESTION TUNE-UP PLAN

Step 1: preparation

First, clear out your cupboards of some of the foods that have a negative effect on your digestive tract. Take my book with you into the kitchen and use it as your "bad-food buster". The following are out: fizzy drinks; white bread, rice and pasta; cream and ice cream; custard; tomato ketchup; pickles; vinegar; instant mashed potatoes; cakes, sugar, sweets, chocolates and biscuits; crisps; margarine, lard and other fats; peanut butter and jams; breakfast cereals; oven chips and microwave meals; pies; dried fruit; heavy yellow cheeses, such as Cheddar; pizza. Replace all these bad foods with the healthy foods that you will need for your meals. Read the menu plan and do a complete shop so that you don't have to worry about any missing ingredients during the plan.

Give your kitchen a spring clean. Take everything off the shelves and throw away any out-of-date foods. If you don't already have a simple steamer (one that you place on top of a pot of boiling water) now is the time to get one. Stock up on some herbal teas, especially chamomile and peppermint, both excellent digestive tonics.

Ask any other members of your household to join you in your new eating plan, especially if you usually do the cooking. And buy a good massage oil for the massage. I suggest your favourite essential oil diluted in grapeseed or apricot oil.

Step 2: menu plan

DAY ONE

Digest:aid juice If you do not have a problem with yeast, sugar or candida: Papaya and pineapple juice (p.104); if you do have a problem with yeast, sugar or candida: Carrot and celery juice (p.105)

Breakfast Warm linseed (flax seed) porridge (p.102)

Lunch Grilled (broiled) mackerel with Thai salad (p.108)

Dinner Spring vegetable frittata (p.111), followed by Mango treat (p.115) for dessert

Before bed Max's soothing digestive tea (p.91)

DAY TWO

Digest:aid juice If you do not have a problem with yeast, sugar or candida: Apricot and grape juice (p.104); if you do have a problem with yeast, sugar or candida: Carrot and celery juice (p.105)

Breakfast Warm linseed (flax seed) porridge (p.102)

Lunch Warm Puy lentil salad with grilled (broiled) chicken (p.109)

Dinner Slow-cooked pumpkin with canellini beans and gremolata (p.112), followed by Mixed berries and papaya (p.114) for dessert

Before bed Max's soothing digestive tea (p.91)

SNACKS

One of the main aims of the digestion plans is to rest your digestive system as much as possible. As a result, you should try to avoid snacks altogether.

Step 3: action

When you exercise your body, you tone up your visible muscles, making your body appear leaner and fitter, and you also tone up your insides. Follow the exercise and stretching advice in Chapter 6 throughout the weekend to ensure that you get the most out of the time you have. In addition, try the following massage.

MASSAGING THE ABDOMEN Our stomachs and intestines are among our most vulnerable areas when it comes to stress and emotional tension – think how knotted your stomach becomes when you feel nervous. We store all kinds of emotional and mental pain in the muscles of the abdomen. When the muscles become tight, blood supply to the gastrointestinal tract reduces, which retards digestive function. A gentle massage (right) can help to release any stored-up tension and restore blood-flow to this sensitive area. Be gentle and start slowly. Don't be surprised if you need a bowel motion after the massage as the strokes relax the large and small intestines, which helps to move the stool along; they also break up the stool, making it easier to pass. In addition massage helps to loosen what naturopaths call the mucous plaque that lines the lower parts of your large intestine. This plaque is caused by the build-up and hardening of the normally slimy mucus that should help your stool to pass easily through the large intestine. When the mucus hardens, it is, of course, less slippery and the stool itself becomes more solid and gets stuck. Abdominal massage, targeted at the bowels, loosens the hardened mucus and so helps the bowels to work better.

ABDOMINAL MASSAGE

During the plan, practise this massage for 10 to 15 minutes twice a day (in the mornings and evenings), while lying on your bed. Always apply light pressure to your abdomen and to any painful areas. If you feel any deep discomfort, stop. Always massage with your whole hand and not just with your fingertips. Dilute your massage oil before you begin (see Step 1: Preparation, opposite).

1 Make sure the room is warm. Take off your top and loosen your skirt or trousers. Lie down and stretch out your legs. Relax. Place your hands on your abdomen so that your fingers lie just above the groin. Listen to the rhythm of your breath and feel the movement of your abdomen as you inhale and exhale. Feel the gentle pressure on your palms as you inhale fully. During the exhalation let your hands vibrate gently. Do this for two minutes.

2 Put some oil on your hands, just enough to help you massage smoothly. Place one hand on top of the other, fingers pointing in opposite directions, and place the lowermost palm on the lower right part of your abdomen. Breathe gently.

3 Press in gently using your whole hand and, in a sweeping motion and applying constant pressure, move up toward your ribs, then across under the ribs to the top left side of your abdomen. Keep pressing in as you move your hands down the left side, stopping at the lower left of your abdomen. Release your hands and relax for a minute, breathing gently.

4 Place your hands on top of each other again and on the right side of your abdomen. Gently draw your hands across to the left side. Stop and then pull your hands back across to the right side. Repeat this kneading motion for a few minutes. Relax and then get up when you are ready.

THE DEEPER DIGESTION TUNE-UP

Fantastic! You have decided to stay in for the long haul and do some great work on your digestion. The following plans cover one and four weeks. Begin with the two days I outline in the weekend plan and get stuck in here with a further five days or three weeks, depending on just how much great work you want to do!

Why should I choose a longer tune-up?

The deeper tune-ups will really turn around your digestion, helping you to remove (and then later identify) which foods upset your system to cause all the symptoms of poor digestion. The benefits can reach well into the long term, perhaps even helping to protect you from diseases such as bowel cancer.

As I have mentioned, one of the factors that causes bloating and intestinal discomfort is food sensitivity (or allergy – a stronger form of sensitivity). Your weekend digestion tune-up should have really helped to reduce your symptoms as it removed most of the common allergenic foods, including wheat, cow's dairy and sugar. Things in your gut should have calmed down and the healing process should now be in full swing. However, if certain foods are causing you trouble, we need a bit longer to identify them. Seven days will give your digestive tract a real rest, making it easier for you to identify which foods, if any, you should not be eating. If, at the end of the week, you are still bloated, uncomfortable or suffering any other signs of allergy, perhaps you are reacting to other foods that are still in your menu plan. Keep writing your food and drink diary (see p.91), making careful note of any symptoms you might have.

What benefits will I achieve?

The idea that you are what you eat has been the basis of naturopathic medicine for the last thousand years. Nevertheless, in reality it's a bit more complicated than that. I think it would be more accurate to say that "you are what you absorb from your food". You might eat only organic, fresh, nutrient-laden food, but you will get no benefit from all that good input if you do not absorb the nutrients. I would estimate that more than 70 per cent of the people who consult me in my clinic have sub-optimal digestion. My feeling is that a week of digestive detox will see a 40 per cent resolution in the common digestive problems I encounter (the bloating, flatulence, diarrhea, constipation and so on), whereas a whole four weeks on the program should see an 80 per cent resolution. Taking the supplements on page 92 will speed up the healing process in the digestive tract and allow some of my clients – and my readers! – to completely overcome all their digestive problems.

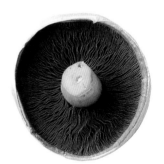 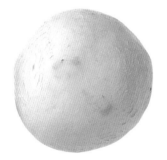 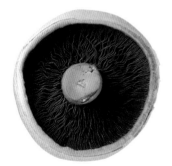

MAX'S MOTIVATOR

WOULDN'T IT BE NICE NOT TO BE ADVERSELY AFFECTED BY FOODS?
Heal your digestive tract now and move to an "indigestion-free zone". After your digestive cleanse, you will probably be able to eat whichever pure foods you like – even the sugary ones! A night out won't end up as a festival of antacids; and a quick snack won't steal your energy. You will feel cleaner, lighter and more toned – on the inside and out. You will look and feel great. What more motivation do you need?

THE ONE-WEEK DIGESTION TUNE-UP PLAN

Step 1: preparation

Do all the things you did for the weekend plan and then can I suggest that you think about the foods that you crave? Chocolate, chips, thick white bread with butter? These are your danger foods. In fact, you may even be allergic or sensitive to them, as a craving often indicates a food allergy. At the very least you are most probably addicted to them. I can hear the denials already. Me? Addicted to certain foods? Madness! Well, addiction is a funny thing. How it works with food is like this. Foods that alter your body's biochemistry in a negative way can be classed as addictive. Some of these changes seem fine, for example the initial boost of energy we get when we have a coffee or a sugary snack. Other changes are slightly more sinister. Take the feeling you might experience after a toasted cheese sandwich, laden with allergenic wheat and cow's dairy (if you are fine with these, that is great, I am just using this as an example). I have clients who feel "stoned" after a hit of an allergenic cheese-and-wheat sandwich. To come back to earth, these clients often need help – usually in the form of an "energizing" coffee. Prepare for this detox by listing, and clearing from your cupboards, all the foods that have a big impact on your energy levels. Just like any recreational drug, the "hit" from these foods is only temporary and energy imbalances will leave you feeling exhausted for most of the day.

Step 2: menu plan

The two days that you have already spent on your digestive tune-up are having a profound effect on your digestion. Over the following five days you are going to optimize its function. To do this we make use of the power that certain fruits and vegetables have to soothe digestion. Best of all, desserts are made up of four of my favourite digestive tonic fruits – papaya, pineapple, mango and pear. The first three have wonderful enzymes in them that help to break down proteins in your digestive tract, reduce inflammation and generally improve the overall health of the bowel lining. You may find that you bloat a little to start with, because of the strong cleansing action of the fruits. Just chew them well and eat small portions, well away from your main course. Pears provide a gentle laxative to soothe away constipation and also help to prevent the growth of bad flora in the intestines.

Warm foods are easier to digest, which is why I suggest a slow-cooked porridge most mornings. Why slow-cooked? Cooking grains for long periods helps your stomach and small intestines to digest them and releases energy quickly into your digestive tract, preparing it for the day ahead.

NOTE: In the following menu plan, use days one and two from the weekend digestive tune-up. See page 98 for Step 3: action for the one-week plan.

THE ONE-WEEK MENU PLAN

DAY 3

Digest:aid juice Apple and pear juice (p.105)

Breakfast Warm linseed (flax seed) porridge (p.102)

Lunch Winter walnut salad (p.108)

Dinner Griddled tuna with pineapple salsa salad (p.111), followed by Papaya and pineapple (p.114) for dessert

Before bed Max's soothing digestive tea (p.91)

DAY 4

Digest:aid juice Carrot and celery juice (p.105)

Breakfast Warm grain and seed porridge (p.102)

Lunch Warm Portobello mushroom, green bean and pumpkin seed salad (p.109)

Dinner Teriyaki salmon with glazed vegetables (p.113), followed by Mango treat (p.115) for dessert

Before bed Max's soothing digestive tea (p.91)

DAY 5

Digest:aid juice Apricot and grape juice (p.104)

Breakfast Warm linseed (flax seed) porridge (p.102)

Lunch Thai-style chicken soup (p.110)

Dinner Chicken with roast carrots, leeks and fennel (p.113), followed by Papaya and pineapple (p.114)

Before bed Max's soothing digestive tea (p.91)

DAY 6

Digest:aid juice Apple and pear juice (p.105)

Breakfast Yummy gluten-free crêpes (p.103)

Lunch Warm Puy lentil salad with grilled (broiled) chicken (p.109)

Dinner Spring vegetable frittata (p.111), followed by Pear with red raspberry sauce (p.115) for dessert

Before bed Max's soothing digestive tea (p.91)

DAY 7

Digest:aid juice Carrot and celery juice (p.105)

Breakfast Bio yogurt crunch (p.103)

Lunch Grilled (broiled) mackerel with Thai salad (p.108)

Dinner Slow-cooked pumpkin with canellini beans and gremolata (p.112), followed by Mixed berries and papaya (p.114)

Before bed Max's soothing digestive tea (p.91)

SNACKS

As with the Weekend Digestion Tune-up Plan, the aim for this week is to rest your digestive tract. As a result, please avoid snacking between your meals.

Step 3: action

Feel free to adjust the following breathing, relaxing, stretching (BRS) schedule to suit your lifestyle, but do aim to do 15 to 20 minutes BRS each day. Have a look at the exercises in Chapter 6 too.

BREATHING Correct abdominal breathing massages all the internal digestive organs and frees up the diaphragm, allowing blood to flow freely, bathing the cells and organs of the digestive tract with fresh, oxygenated blood. Not a bad bonus for correct breathing. I suggest doing the breathing technique on the right every morning.

RELAXING As you now know, a good blood supply to the stomach and intestines ensures the healthy production of digestive enzymes. Take a few deep, relaxing breaths before, during and after each meal or snack to release the knotted-up tension that hampers blood-flow. In addition, the progressive muscular relaxation (PMR) technique on page 225 aims to take the tightness out of your stomach, again freeing up your circulation. Try to do the PMR routine every day last thing at night, or whenever you start to feel stress building up during the day.

STRETCHING Stretching improves blood-flow to your bowels and energizes you for the day ahead. The upward stretch on the right helps to activate the digestive tract and promote good digestion and elimination by massaging all of the internal digestive organs. This is the perfect stretch to do before eating, as it wakes up your internal organs and prepares the stomach to meet your meal.

ABDOMINAL BREATHING INTERNAL MASSAGE

1 Stand with your feet shoulder-width apart. Lean forward and place your hands on your knees. Exhale gently.

2 Keeping your breath relaxed and even, drop your chin down toward your chest (you can place your hands on your thighs if it is easier). Relax.

3 Inhale and push out your abdomen. Exhale and pull in your abdomen, pulling in your belly button toward your spine. Repeat the pushing and pulling slowly nine more times, taking care not to hyperventilate. Stand up slowly. You may feel light-headed after this exercise so have a chair nearby to sit on.

DIGESTIVE UPWARD STRETCH

1 Stand up straight with your feet shoulder-width apart. Fix your gaze on an object or point on the wall directly in front of your eyes. Interlace your fingers.

2 Breathe in. Raise your arms overhead, keeping your fingers interlaced, and turning your palms so that they end facing upward. Look up at your hands.

3 Lift your heels and soles of your feet as though you are being drawn upward. Stretch your body. Exhale and slowly return your heels to the ground. Drop your arms to your sides. Repeat the stretch ten times.

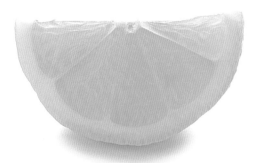

EXTENDING THE PLAN TO FOUR WEEKS

Three more weeks might seem like an age to be on a healthy-eating plan. The funny thing is that after completing the following weeks, you will most probably never return to your old eating habits.

Preparing, Eating and BRS

Use the weekend and week-long preparation guidelines to prepare for the following three weeks. Follow the eating plan on pages 100–101. By all means adjust it to your preferences, but do try to keep a good variety in your diet. You could add a few more herbs to the recipes if you like – ginger, coriander and rosemary are all great for digestion. In addition to daily stretching and breathing techniques (see opposite), follow the advice on exercising on pages 214–16. Regular exercise helps to normalize your bowel motions by massaging and stretching the bowels, and reduces stress to improve blood-flow to the digestive organs and ensure the proper production of digestive enzymes.

Turbo-boost your digestive recovery

Certain fruits, herbs and vegetables work to tone up and heal your digestive tract, and include: chicory, endive (escarole), radicchio, dandelion leaves and dandelion root. These bitter medicinal plants make excellent digestive tonics – although the taste of them can take a bit of getting used to! During the four-week plan, try one or two tonic-only days. Juice any combination of the above list of plants and drink the juice throughout the day. At the end of the day have a cup of my soothing digestive tea (see p.91).

NOTE If you suffer from diabetes or are on medication of any sort, do not do juice-only days without consulting your health professional first.

THE FOUR-WEEK DIGESTION TUNE-UP MENU PLAN

Use the menu plans from the weekend and week digestion tune-ups for your first week; here are the menu plans for weeks two to four. Begin each day with a digestive juice (see pp.104–107) and end each day with the digestive tea (see p.91). Rules on snacks and desserts apply as they did for the shorter tune-up plans: snacks are off the menu, and for desserts stock up on those fantastic digestive enzymes found in the dessert recipes on pages 114–15. Feel free to juggle the recipes according to your preference, but try to keep the sense of variety.

WEEK TWO

DAY	BREAKFAST	LUNCH	DINNER
Monday	Warm linseed (flax seed) porridge (p.102)	Grilled (broiled) mackerel with Thai salad (p.108)	Spring vegetable frittata (p.111)
Tuesday	Warm grain and seed porridge (p.102)	Warm Portobello mushroom, green bean and pumpkin seed salad (p.109)	Teriyaki salmon with glazed vegetables (p.113)
Wednesday	Yummy gluten-free crêpes (p.103)	Winter walnut salad (p.108)	Slow-cooked pumpkin with canellini beans and gremolata (p.112)
Thursday	Bio yogurt crunch (p.103)	Warm Puy lentil salad with grilled (broiled) chicken (p.109)	Griddled tuna with pineapple salsa salad (p.111)
Friday	Warm linseed (flax seed) porridge (p.102)	Thai-style chicken soup (p.110)	Teriyaki salmon with glazed vegetables (p.113)
Saturday	Warm grain and seed porridge (p.102)	Grilled mackerel with Thai salad (p.108)	Chicken breast with roast carrots, leeks and fennel (p.113)
Sunday	Yummy gluten-free crêpes (p.103)	Winter walnut salad (p.108)	Spring vegetable frittata (p.111)

WEEK THREE

DAY	BREAKFAST	LUNCH	DINNER
Monday	Bio yogurt crunch (p.103)	Thai-style chicken soup (p.110)	Griddled tuna with pineapple salsa salad (p.111)
Tuesday	Warm linseed (flax seed) porridge (p.102)	Warm Puy lentil salad with grilled (broiled) chicken (p.109)	Spring vegetable frittata (p.111)
Wednesday	Warm grain and seed porridge (p.102)	Warm Portobello mushroom, green bean and pumpkin seed salad (p.109)	Chicken with roast carrots, leeks and fennel (p.113)
Thursday	Yummy gluten-free crêpes (p.103)	Grilled (broiled) mackerel with Thai salad (p.108)	Griddled tuna with pineapple salsa salad (p.111)
Friday	Bio yogurt crunch (p.103)	Thai-style chicken soup (p.110)	Slow-cooked pumpkin with canellini beans and gremolata (p.112)
Saturday	Warm linseed (flax seed) porridge (p.102)	Warm Portobello mushroom, green bean and pumpkin seed salad (p.109)	Teriyaki salmon with glazed vegetables (p.113)
Sunday	Warm grain and seed porridge (p.102)	Warm Puy lentil salad with grilled (broiled) chicken (p.109)	Spring vegetable frittata (p.111)

WEEK FOUR

DAY	BREAKFAST	LUNCH	DINNER
Monday	Yummy gluten-free crêpes (p.103)	Winter walnut salad (p.108)	Chicken with roast carrots, leeks and fennel (p.113)
Tuesday	Bio yogurt crunch (p.103)	Grilled (broiled) mackerel with Thai-style salad (p.108)	Slow-cooked pumpkin with canellini beans and gremolata (p.112)
Wednesday	Warm linseed (flax seed) porridge (p.102)	Warm Portobello mushroom, green bean and pumpkin seed salad (p.109)	Griddled tuna with pineapple salsa salad (p.111)
Thursday	Warm grain and seed porridge (p.102)	Warm Puy lentil salad with grilled (broiled) chicken (p.109)	Teriyaki salmon with glazed vegetables (p.113)
Friday	Yummy gluten-free crêpes (p.103)	Thai-style chicken soup (p.110)	Spring vegetable frittata (p.111)
Saturday	Bio yogurt crunch (p.103)	Warm Portobello mushroom, green bean and pumpkin seed salad (p.109)	Griddled tuna with pineapple salsa salad (p.111)
Sunday	Warm linseed (flax seed) porridge (p.102)	Grilled (broiled) mackerel with Thai-style salad (p.108)	Chicken with roast carrots, leeks and fennel (p.113)

DIGESTION BREAKFASTS

Warm linseed (flax seed) porridge

SERVES 1
PREPARATION TIME 5 MINUTES
COOKING TIME 30 MINUTES

50g/2oz/1 cup grain (Choose from either rolled oats, rolled quinoa, rolled rice or rolled millet. Use only one grain. If you are allergic to oats, please use the rolled quinoa or millet.)

Soya (soy), goat's or sheep's milk as necessary

1 heaped tsp fresh linseeds (flax seeds), ground

1 tbsp live culture goat's or sheep's yogurt

1 heaped tbsp fresh berries (such as blueberries, raspberries and blackberries)

Ground cinnamon (optional)

1 Place the grain in a large bowl and cover it with water. Soak it overnight in the refrigerator.

2 Slow cook the grain on a low heat for a minimum of 30 minutes (ideally an hour), adding milk as necessary to achieve a thick, smooth consistency.

3 Take the porridge off the heat and stir in the linseeds (flax seeds), yogurt and berries.

4 Stir in the cinnamon to taste, and serve.

Warm grain and seed porridge

SERVES 1
PREPARATION TIME 5 MINUTES
COOKING TIME 30 MINUTES

50g/2oz/1 cup grain (Choose from rolled oats, rolled rice, rolled quinoa or rolled millet. Use only one grain. If you are allergic to oats please use the rolled quinoa or millet.)

Soya (soy), goat's or sheep's milk as necessary

1 heaped tsp fresh sunflower, pumpkin and sesame seeds (ground)

1 tbsp live culture goat's or sheep's yogurt

½ ripe pear, mashed

Ground cinnamon or nutmeg to taste

1 Place the grain in a large bowl and cover with water. Soak it overnight in the refrigerator.

2 Slow cook the grain on a low heat for a minimum of 30 minutes (an hour is ideal), adding milk as necessary.

3 Remove the porridge from the heat and stir in the seeds, yogurt and pear.

4 Add the cinnamon or nutmeg to taste.

Yummy gluten-free crêpes

MAKES 5 PANCAKES
PREPARATION TIME 10 MINUTES
COOKING TIME 10 MINUTES

100g/3½oz/1 cup brown rice flour
3 fresh, organic, free-range eggs
55–110ml/2–3 fl oz/¼–½ cup water
1½ tbsp cold-pressed sunflower oil
Lemon juice/chopped banana/100% maple syrup to serve

1   Mix together the brown rice flour, eggs and oil in a bowl.

2   Slowly add the water to the rice mixture and mix until smooth.

3   Lightly oil a frying pan (skillet) and then heat the pan on the stove. Pour in a small amount of batter and cook each side until golden brown.

4   Serve the pancakes plain, or with a squeeze of lemon, some chopped banana, or 100-per-cent maple syrup.

Bio yogurt crunch

SERVES 1
PREPARATION TIME 5 MINUTES
COOKING TIME 5 MINUTES

1 tsp sunflower seeds
1 tsp pine nuts
1 ripe pear
1 small cup live yogurt (cow's, goat's, soya [soy] or sheep's)
1 tsp linseeds (flax seeds), ground

1   Gently dry-fry the sunflower seeds and pine nuts until they are a very light brown in colour. Take care not to burn the seeds. Remove the seeds from the pan and set aside.

2   Mash the pear and fold it into the yogurt, then mix in the linseeds (flax seeds).

3   Pour the yogurt mixture into a bowl and sprinkle the dry-fried seeds over the top to serve.

DIGESTION JUICES

Papaya and pineapple juice

SERVES 1
PREPARATION TIME 5 MINUTES

1 ripe papaya
1 large slice ripe pineapple
1 large carrot
1 stick of celery
1 tsp fresh lemon juice

1   Juice the carrot, pineapple and celery.

2   Blend with the mashed papaya and add the lemon.

3   Pour into a glass and sip slowly, mixing with your saliva to help to digest the juice.

Apricot and grape juice

SERVES 1
PREPARATION TIME 5 MINUTES

2 ripe apricots
10 seedless green grapes
½ head of cabbage
1 carrot

1   Juice the cabbage, grapes and carrot.

2   Blend the apricots and stir into the juice.

3   Pour into a glass and sip slowly, mixing with your saliva.

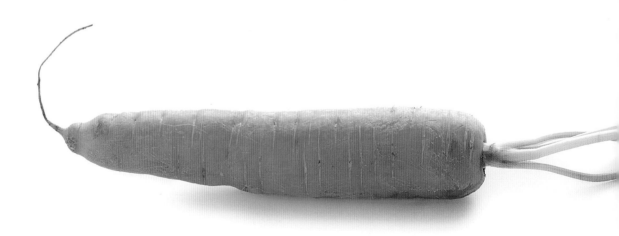

Apple and pear juice

SERVES 1
PREPARATION TIME 5 MINUTES

1 green apple
1 slice pineapple
1 small carrot
1 small beetroot (beet)
⅓ of a cucumber
3 leaves spinach
1 pear
1 peach
1 ripe apricot

1 Juice the apple, pineapple, carrot, beetroot (beet), cucumber and spinach.

2 Blend the pear, peach and apricot, and mix with the juice.

3 Pour into a glass and sip slowly, mixing with your saliva.

Carrot and celery juice

SERVES 1
PREPARATION TIME 5 MINUTES

2 carrots
1 stick celery
1 fennel bulb
4 leaves kale
Ginger to taste

1 Juice the carrots, celery, fennel, kale and ginger.

2 Pour into a glass and sip slowly, mixing with your saliva.

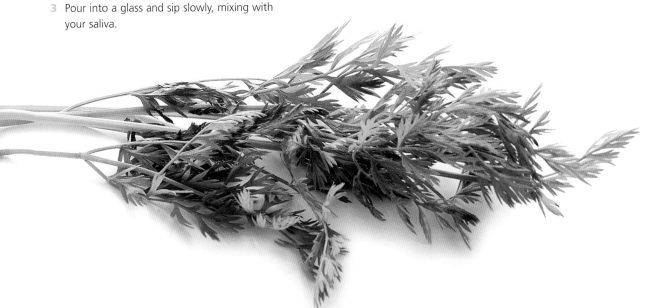

Carrot and grape juice

SERVES 1
PREPARATION TIME 5 MINUTES

15 green, seedless grapes
1 large carrot
3 leaves spinach
Juice of half a lemon
Juice of 1 orange

1 Juice the grapes, carrot and spinach.

2 Add the fresh orange and lemon juice.

3 Pour into a glass and sip slowly, mixing with your saliva to begin the digestive process in the mouth.

Red pear juice

SERVES 1
PREPARATION TIME 5 MINUTES

Small handful basil leaves
1 medium beetroot (beet), cut into chunks
1 carrot, cut into chunks
2 ripe pears
Juice of 1 lime

1 Roll up the individual basil leaves tightly. Begin juicing the beetroot (beet) and carrot, chunks at a time, occasionally adding in a rolled-up basil leaf to help the basil pass through the juicer.

2 Add the lime juice.

3 Pour into a glass and sip slowly, mixing with your saliva.

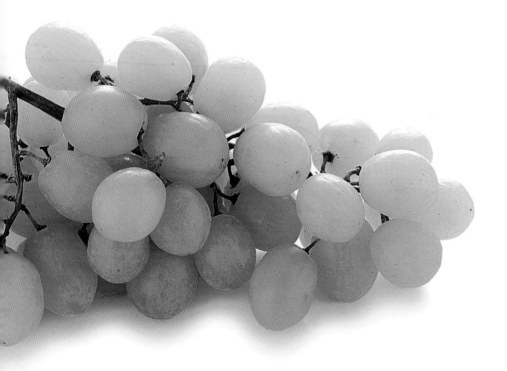
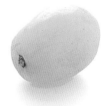

Carrot and pineapple juice

SERVES 1
PREPARATION TIME 5 MINUTES

2 large carrots
1 large slice pineapple
1 tbsp live goat's yogurt

1 Juice the carrots and pineapple.

2 Stir in the yogurt.

3 Pour into a glass and sip slowly, mixing with your saliva.

Lemon and papaya juice

SERVES 1
PREPARATION TIME 5 MINUTES

1 ripe papaya, deskinned and pips removed
2 tbsp live goat's or sheep's yogurt
1 ripe banana

1 Blend all the ingredients together.

2 Pour into a glass and sip slowly, mixing with your saliva.

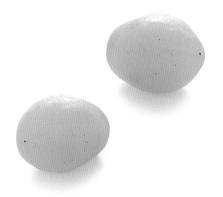
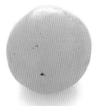
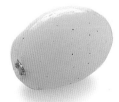

DIGESTION LUNCHES

Winter walnut salad

SERVES 2
PREPARATION TIME 10 MINUTES
COOKING TIME 15 MINUTES

1 large radicchio head (200g/7oz), cut into 8 wedges
(if you can't find radicchio, use chicory)

1 large firm pear, core removed and cut into
8 lengthways

1 tbsp extra virgin olive oil

2 handfuls lamb's lettuce (40g/1½oz)

50g/2oz walnut pieces, lightly toasted

3 tbsp walnut oil

1 tbsp cider vinegar

1 Preheat a griddle pan. Brush the radicchio and
pear wedges with the olive oil. Griddle the
radicchio for 3 minutes on each side, until
wilted. Griddle the pear for 4 minutes on each
side, until starting to soften.

2 Arrange the radicchio, pear and lettuce on two
plates and scatter over the walnut pieces.

3 Whisk together the walnut oil and vinegar in a
small bowl and drizzle over the salad before
serving.

Grilled (broiled) mackerel with Thai salad

SERVES 2
PREPARATION TIME 15 MINUTES
COOKING TIME 6 MINUTES

2 x 110g/4oz mackerel fillets

1 medium green apple, cored and cut into matchsticks

6 salad onions, trimmed and finely sliced

Small bunch coriander (cilantro), leaves only

Small bunch mint, leaves roughly torn

Small bunch basil, leaves roughly torn

2 tbsp lime juice

1 tsp fresh ginger, grated

2 lime quarters, to serve

1 Preheat the grill (broiler) to high and grill (broil)
the mackerel for 2–3 minutes on each side, until
cooked through.

2 Put the apple, onions and herbs in a large bowl.
Whisk the lime juice and ginger together in a
small bowl, pour over the salad and toss gently.

3 Divide the salad between two plates and top
each with a mackerel fillet. Serve with the lime
quarters.

Warm Portobello mushroom, green bean and pumpkin seed salad

SERVES 2
PREPARATION TIME 15 MINUTES
COOKING TIME 10 MINUTES

3 large Portobello mushrooms, each cut into 8 wedges

3 tbsp extra virgin olive oil

2 medium cloves garlic, peeled and crushed

4 sprigs thyme, leaves chopped

Finely grated zest of ½ unwaxed lemon, plus 1 tsp juice

170g/6oz green beans, trimmed

2 tbsp pumpkin seeds, lightly toasted (if you don't have pumpkin seed oil, use an additional 1 tbsp of extra virgin olive oil)

1 tbsp pumpkin seed oil, to serve

1   Preheat the grill (broiler) to high. Put the mushrooms, 2 tbsp olive oil, garlic, thyme and lemon zest in a large bowl and mix well. Grill (broil) for 8–9 minutes, turning 2–3 times, until the mushrooms are cooked through.

2   Put a large pan of water on to boil. Cook the beans in boiling water for 3 minutes until just tender. Drain.

3   Put the mushrooms and beans in a large bowl. Whisk the remaining olive oil and the lemon juice together in a small bowl and pour over the salad. Toss well, divide between two plates and scatter over the pumpkin seeds. Drizzle over the pumpkin seed oil to serve.

Warm Puy lentil salad with grilled (broiled) chicken

SERVES 2
PREPARATION TIME 15 MINUTES
COOKING TIME 30 MINUTES

110g/4oz/⅗ cup Puy lentils, rinsed

1 bay leaf

2 sprigs thyme

Small bunch flat leaf parsley, chopped, 5 stalks reserved

600ml/20 fl oz/2½ cups water plus 3 tbsp

½ small red onion, peeled and finely chopped

1 large stick celery, finely sliced

1 large handful asparagus tips (90g/3oz), trimmed and cut into 5mm/¼in pieces

2 tbsp extra virgin olive oil

1 tbsp lemon juice

2 x 110g/4oz skinless, boneless organic chicken breasts

2 lemon quarters, to serve.

1   Put the lentils, bay leaf, thyme, parsley stalks and 600ml/20 fl oz/2½ cups water in a saucepan. Place over a medium heat, cover and simmer for 20 minutes, until the lentils are tender. Drain and discard the herbs. Transfer to a large bowl.

2   Put the onion, celery, asparagus, 1 tbsp olive oil and 3 tbsp water in a 20cm/8in frying pan (skillet). Place over a medium-low heat and cook for 10 minutes. Stir into the lentils with the remaining olive oil, lemon juice and parsley.

3   Preheat the grill (broiler) to medium. Put the chicken breasts between two large pieces of greaseproof paper and use a rolling pin to flatten the breasts into escalopes 1cm/½in thick. Grill (broil) for 5–6 minutes on each side.

4   Divide the lentil salad between two plates and top with the chicken. Serve with lemon quarters.

Thai-style chicken soup

SERVES 2
PREPARATION TIME 20 MINUTES
COOKING TIME 45 MINUTES

2 medium shallots (scallions), peeled and finely sliced

2 medium cloves garlic, peeled and finely sliced

2 sticks lemongrass, roughly chopped

2 tsp fresh ginger, grated

6 black peppercorns

Zest of 1 unwaxed lime, pared with a potato peeler, plus 2 tbsp juice

Small bunch coriander (cilantro), chopped, reserve stalks

½ fresh red chilli, deseeded and finely chopped (for medium heat)

1.2 litres/40 fl oz/5 cups water

2 x 110g/4oz skinless, boneless organic chicken breasts

4 salad onions, trimmed and finely sliced

1 small carrot, peeled and cut into matchsticks

Handful baby corn (85g/3oz), cut into 4 lengthways

2 small handfuls mange tout (85g/3oz), cut into matchsticks

2 lime quarters, to serve

1 Put the shallots (scallions), garlic, lemongrass, ginger, peppercorns, lime zest and coriander (cilantro) stalks, and half the chilli in a large saucepan and add the water. Place over a medium heat and simmer for 15 minutes.

2 Add the chicken breasts and cook for a further 20 minutes, turning the chicken over halfway through.

3 Put the onions, chopped coriander (cilantro), remaining chilli and lime juice in a small bowl and mix. Leave to stand for 10 minutes.

4 Remove the chicken breasts from the saucepan and strain the stock through a fine sieve into a bowl or jug. Shred the chicken and put back into the saucepan, add the strained stock and place over a medium heat. Add the carrot and baby corn and simmer for 2 minutes. Add the mange tout and cook for a further 2 minutes, until just cooked.

5 Ladle the soup into two large bowls. Spoon over the coriander (cilantro) and lime mixture and serve with the lime quarters.

DIGESTION DINNERS

Griddled tuna with pineapple salsa salad

SERVES 2
PREPARATION TIME 20 MINUTES
COOKING TIME 5 MINUTES

½ medium pineapple (400g/14oz), quartered, cored and skin removed and finely sliced
¼ medium cucumber (110g/4oz), halved and finely sliced
Small bunch coriander (cilantro), leaves only
8 salad onions, trimmed and finely sliced
½ fresh red chilli, finely chopped (for medium heat)
2 tbsp extra virgin olive oil
4 tsp lemon juice
2 x 150g/5oz line-caught yellow fin tuna steaks, cut 5cm/2in thick
2 lime quarters, to serve

1 Put the pineapple, cucumber, coriander (cilantro), onions and chilli in a large bowl. Whisk the olive oil and lemon juice together in a small bowl. Pour over the salad and toss well.

2 Preheat a griddle pan. Griddle the tuna for 1 minute (rare) or 2 minutes (medium-rare) on each side.

3 Divide the salad between two plates and top with the tuna. Serve with the lime quarters.

Spring vegetable frittata

SERVES 2
PREPARATION TIME 15 MINUTES
COOKING TIME 20 MINUTES

Large handful asparagus tips (110g/4oz), trimmed with stalks cut into 1cm/½in pieces
2 handfuls podded young broad beans (60g/2oz)
6 large organic, free-range eggs
2 tsp lemon juice
8 large leaves basil, shredded
6–8 morel mushrooms, halved (use quartered chestnut mushrooms if morels are unavailable)
1 tbsp extra virgin olive oil
4 salad onions, trimmed and finely sliced
1 medium clove garlic, peeled and crushed

1 Bring a large pan of water to the boil. Add the beans and asparagus and cook for 2 minutes, then drain and rinse under a cold tap until cool.

2 Put the eggs, lemon juice and basil in a small bowl and whisk well to combine.

3 Put the mushrooms and olive oil in a deep 20cm/8in non-stick frying pan (skillet) over a high heat and stir-fry for 5 minutes. Reduce the heat to low and add the onions, garlic, asparagus and beans. Cook for 1 minute. Pour the eggs into the pan and cook for 7–8 minutes until the base of the frittata is set and the top is a little runny.

4 Preheat the grill (broiler) to medium and grill (broil) the top of the frittata for 2 minutes. Ease the frittata onto a large plate and cut into wedges. Serve with a finely chopped green salad.

Slow-cooked pumpkin with canellini beans and gremolata

SERVES 2
PREPARATION TIME 30 MINUTES (PLUS OVERNIGHT SOAKING)
COOKING TIME 2 HOURS AND 10 MINUTES (INCLUDES 1 HOUR COOKING TIME FOR BEANS)

170g/6oz/1 cup canellini beans

1 small onion, peeled and chopped

1 large stick celery, chopped

2 medium cloves garlic, peeled, one crushed and one chopped

2 tbsp extra virgin olive oil

2 sprigs thyme, chopped

2 sprigs oregano, chopped

340g/12oz/2½ cups pumpkin, cut into 2.5cm/1in cubes (you can use butternut or acorn squash as an alternative, if you like)

100ml/3½ fl oz/½ cup vegetable stock

Finely grated zest of 1 unwaxed lemon, plus 4 tsp juice

1 small bunch flat leaf parsley, finely chopped

40g/1½oz watercress

1 Soak the beans overnight and cook according to the packet instructions. Drain the beans.

2 Put the onion, celery, crushed garlic and 1 tbsp olive oil in a medium cast-iron casserole dish. Place over a low heat, cover and cook very gently for 20 minutes. Stir occasionally to prevent the vegetables from catching on the bottom of the pan.

3 Add the thyme, oregano, pumpkin, beans and vegetable stock. Re-cover and continue to cook gently for 40 minutes. Uncover the pot and simmer for 10 minutes, until the pumpkin and beans are tender and most of the stock has been absorbed. Stir in 2 tsp lemon juice.

4 Make the gremolata while the pumpkin is cooking. Put the parsley, chopped garlic and lemon zest in a small bowl and mix well.

5 Put the watercress in a large bowl. Whisk the remaining olive oil and lemon juice together in a small bowl. Pour over the watercress and toss well.

6 Spoon the pumpkin into two large bowls and sprinkle over the gremolata. Serve the pumpkin with the watercress salad on the side.

Teriyaki salmon with glazed vegetables

SERVES 2
PREPARATION TIME 10 MINUTES
COOKING TIME 15 MINUTES

6 tbsp fresh orange juice

2 tbsp wheat-free tamari

1 tsp fresh ginger, grated

2 x 170g/6oz salmon fillets, skin on

1 tsp extra virgin olive oil

2 medium carrots, cut into matchsticks

2 large handfuls mange tout (170g/6oz)

2 tbsp water

8 salad onions, trimmed and finely sliced

1 Begin by making the teriyaki glaze. Put the orange juice, tamari and ginger in a small saucepan over a high heat. Bring to a rapid boil and cook for 30 seconds, until slightly thickened. Remove from the heat.

2 Preheat the grill (broiler) to high. Grill (broil) the skin side of the salmon for 4–5 minutes, then turn and brush the flesh sides with the teriyaki glaze. Grill for 3 minutes, then brush with glaze again and cook for a further 4–5 minutes, until the salmon is cooked through. Keep warm.

3 Put the olive oil in a wok over a high heat. Add the carrot, mange tout and water and stir-fry for 4 minutes. Add the onions and remaining teriyaki glaze and cook for 1 minute. Divide the vegetables between two plates and top with the salmon.

Chicken with roast carrots, leeks and fennel

SERVES 2
PREPARATION TIME 15 MINUTES
COOKING TIME 50 MINUTES

1 handful baby carrots (110g/4oz), peeled and sliced in half lengthways

4–6 baby leeks, trimmed

Small bulb fennel (200g/7oz), cut into 8 wedges

1 tbsp extra virgin olive oil

2 tbsp water

2 x 250g/9oz organic chicken breast quarters, skin on

1 tsp lemon juice

4 sprigs tarragon, chopped

1 Preheat the oven to 200°C/fan 180°C/400°F/ gas 6.

2 Put the carrots, leeks and fennel in a small roasting pan and sprinkle over the oil and water. Roast at the top of the oven for 10 minutes.

3 Turn the vegetables over in the pan and lay the chicken on top. Return to the oven for 35–40 minutes, until the chicken is cooked through.

4 Put the chicken pieces on two plates and remove the skin to reduce the fat content. Add the lemon juice and tarragon to the roasting pan and toss to coat the vegetables. Transfer the vegetables to the plates and spoon over the pan juices.

NOTE: If you can't get baby vegetables, use ordinary carrots cut into index-finger size pieces and ordinary leeks cut in half lengthways. If you are using boneless chicken breasts, they will take only 25–30 minutes to cook, so allow the vegetables to cook for 20 minutes before adding the chicken.

DIGESTION DESSERTS

Papaya and pineapple

SERVES 1
PREPARATION TIME 5 MINUTES

½ small ripe papaya, sliced
½ small ripe mango, chopped
1 tbsp plain, live culture goat's or sheep's yogurt
½ tsp crushed sunflower seeds
Fresh lime juice to taste

1 Place the papaya and mango in a bowl.

2 Add the yogurt and crushed sunflower seeds.

3 Add a dash of fresh lime juice to taste.

Mixed berries and papaya

SERVES 1
PREPARATION TIME 5 MINUTES

Large handful mixed fresh berries, such as blueberries, raspberries and blackberries
¼ small ripe papaya, chopped
1 tbsp plain, live culture goat's or sheep's yogurt
½ teaspoon of crushed sesame seeds
Fresh orange juice to taste

1 In a small bowl crush the fresh berries with the back of a spoon. Transfer to a larger bowl and mix with the papaya.

2 Add the yogurt and crushed sesame seeds.

3 Add a dash of fresh orange juice to taste.

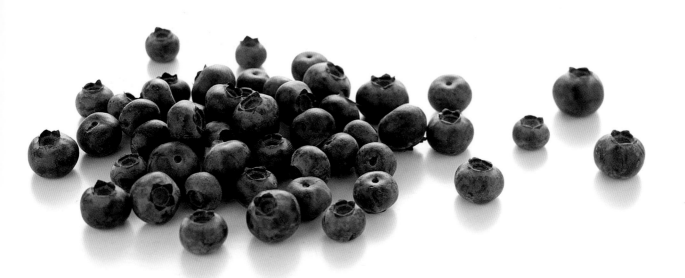

Mango treat

SERVES 1
PREPARATION TIME 5 MINUTES

1 ripe mango
2 tbsp live culture goat's, cow's or sheep's yogurt (use cow's yogurt only if you are not sensitive to it)
1 tsp fresh lemon juice
Pinch freshly ground nutmeg
10 black grapes, cut in half

1 Blend the mango, live yogurt, lemon juice and nutmeg until a smooth purée. Place in a bowl.

2 Garnish with the halved black grapes.

Pear with red raspberry sauce

SERVES 1
PREPARATION TIME 10 MINUTES
COOKING TIME 25 MINUTES

1 large ripe pear
½ cup fresh orange juice (use a ripe, sweet orange)
½ cup fresh raspberries (or blueberries or cherries), puréed
Pinch cinnamon or nutmeg
2.5cm/1in vanilla pod, cracked or sliced down the side
1 sprig fresh mint to garnish

1 Preheat the oven to 240°C/fan 220°C/475°F/ gas 9.

2 Cut the pear in half lengthways, remove the seeds, and core.

3 Place the pear halves cut side down on an oven-proof baking dish.

4 Combine the orange juice, puréed raspberries, cinnamon and vanilla pod, then pour this mixture over the pear halves. Cover the baking dish with tin (aluminum) foil.

5 Place the pear halves in the oven and bake them until they are soft (about 25 minutes).

6 Remove the vanilla pod and place the pear halves cut side up on a plate. Spoon the remaining sauce from the baking tray over the pear. Garnish with a fresh mint leaf.

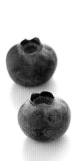

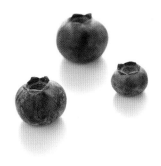

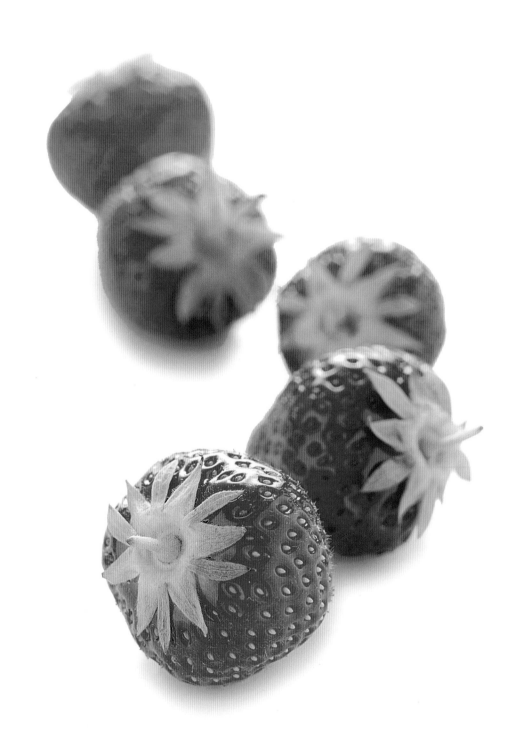

the energy-boost plans

make use of the amazing power of pure foods
to energize you

DO YOU NEED TO INVIGORATE YOUR BODY AND MIND?

ARE YOU:

feeling irritable, stressed and restless?

suffering from low libido?

feeling low in energy?

feeling tired and lethargic?

not sleeping well?

waking unrefreshed?

feeling disinterested in life?

feeling down and depressed?

finding it hard to motivate yourself?

If you answered yes to any of these questions, then this might just be
the most important chapter in a book that you will ever read. You
might be in need of a total energy overhaul using pure foods.

ENERGY MAKES THE WORLD GO ROUND

Without energy our lives are flat and bland, filled with physical and emotional lows and devoid of the sparkle and colour that make life a joy. Energy production is a biochemical process requiring a number of essential nutrients. We need vitamins, minerals, water, carbohydrates, proteins, fats and enzymes to generate energy in our body. If these are missing from our diet, the odds are that we will feel tired and lethargic.

How do we make energy?

Carbohydrates in our foods supply the body with the energy it needs to function. These are found mainly in grains, fruits and vegetables and in smaller amounts in dairy products, but they are divided into two different kinds of carbohydrate: simple and complex.

SIMPLE CARBOHYDRATES These include glucose, table sugar and fruit sugar (fructose), and they release energy quickly into the blood stream, giving a short, sharp energy burst. The energy we get from chocolate, for example, is simple-carbohydrate energy.

COMPLEX CARBOHYDRATES These release sugars slowly into the blood, enabling the body to enjoy a sustained energy output. They are made up of long chains of glucose that are bound together, and are found mainly in wholegrain foods, such as brown rice and rolled oats.

In the body carbohydrates are broken down into blood glucose, which is a major fuel for all of the cells in your body and is the only source of fuel for the brain and the red blood cells. The amount of sugar in the blood needs to be constant to allow you to function with optimum energy throughout the day. Low blood sugars equate to low energy – at the most extreme end of the scale, if your blood sugars fall too low you end up in a coma. So, because blood sugars are so important, a vast array of nutrients are required to facilitate the breakdown and metabolism of glucose. The list of crucial nutrients includes the minerals chromium, zinc and magnesium, and the B-vitamins.

A healthy body, with a full quotient of essential nutrients, will have plenty of energy to maintain health and to govern all of the internal energy-production processes efficiently. So why might this not happen?

What can go wrong?

STRESS AND ADRENAL FUNCTION The quality of your energy and the regulation of blood sugars is partly governed by your adrenal glands. These two amazing little endocrine glands sit above the kidneys and are responsible for producing, among other hormones, adrenaline (epinephrine). In stressful or dangerous situations, adrenaline is produced in large amounts and triggers the fight-or-flight response. Our blood pressure goes up and glucose enters the blood, which pours into the arms, legs and head so that we can fight, run and think. The response is a primitive one – it was originally intended to save us from marauding animals and angry enemies – but these days, for most people at least, this adrenaline-fuelled burst of energy occurs in response to the minor irritations and stresses of daily life. And this is where the problems start.

Relationship or work problems, family pressures and so on might be unwelcome, but they are not life-threatening. Nevertheless, our body responds as though they are, pumping out adrenaline unnecessarily. The overworked adrenal glands eventually become tired and, among other things, adrenaline production slows down. The signs of adrenal exhaustion should be familiar – restless sleep, waking in the early hours, night sweats, poor digestion, blood-pressure problems, blood-sugar fluctuations, fluid retention and dry skin. Tired adrenals have a major impact on your ability to produce and sustain energy.

FOOD ALLERGIES AND FOOD SENSITIVITIES Food sensitivities contribute enormously to modern levels of fatigue. They occur when your immune system overreacts and incorrectly identifies the food that you are eating as a potential invasion by an antigen (see p.84).

A food allergy is a far more serious problem than a sensitivity. In an allergy the immune system reacts potently to a food, with swelling, inflammation and even possible death. Food sensitivities, though, are not life-threatening, and exhibit milder signs, such as tiredness after eating, bloating in the lower abdomen and strong cravings for certain foods. A good way to get a sense of how food allergies or sensitivities can affect you is to think how you feel when your body prepares to fight off flu. Imagine the tiredness, the aches and pains, the heavy head. These symptoms are similar to the symptoms of food sensitivity or allergy – and they occur every time you eat that particular food.

THE SILENT CRY FOR WATER You are 70 per cent water. If you are dehydrated, the chemical processes in your body that require water slow down, and you feel tired. A loss of 2 per cent of water from your body (just 1kg/2lb for a 50kg/110lb person) reduces physical and mental performance by up to a significant 20 per cent. Pure foods contain plenty of water (watermelon contains up to 80 per cent water!). It's time to rehydrate your body and release all that locked-in energy.

THE GLYCEMIC INDEX This is a system of categorizing foods according to their energy output. Carbohydrates (pasta, bread, potatoes, rice, oats, rye and so on) can be classified as low-, medium- or high-GI. The low- and medium-GI foods release energy, in the form of sugar, into the blood at a steady rate, which is good for you. High-GI foods dump sugar very quickly into the blood, creating blood-sugar imbalances and weight gain, as the excess sugars are stored as fat. Take a chocolate bar. The sugar from the chocolate enters your blood stream quickly and raises your blood sugars fast, giving a sense of energy. However, this quick release raises blood sugars far too high. To get rid of the excess sugars, the pancreas releases lots of insulin, but this puts away too much blood sugar, creating a blood-sugar slump. Your energy falls and you reach for another chocolate bar – and so the cycle goes on. Look at the good- and bad-GI foods chart opposite and banish the bad ones from your diet.

THE GI "GOODIES" AND "BADDIES"

TOP GOOD GI FOODS

These are the best examples of foods that support normal blood-sugar levels and good, sustained energy levels.

Apples, berries, rhubarb, tangerines, dried apricots, guavas, lemons, limes, prunes, peaches, pears, plums, grapefruits, cherries

Barley

Legumes (lentils, beans and so on)

Nuts (almonds, walnuts, soy nuts)

Oatmeal

Green peas

Tomatoes

Plain, unsweetened sheep's or goat's yogurt

TOP BAD GI FOODS

These foods can produce high blood-sugar levels and so a high insulin response. These foods leave you depleted of energy a short while after eating them.

Sweets (candy), and any other products containing simple sugars

Fizzy (carbonated) drinks

Biscuits (cookies)

Chocolates

Cakes

Juices with added sugar

Crisps (potato chips) and fries

Sweetened breakfast cereals

White bread

White rice (all types)

White pasta

White flour products

NOTE: The fruits listed below are high GI, but if the choice is between a chocolate biscuit and a high-GI fruit, the fruit wins every time.

Banana

Watermelon

Cantaloupe melon

Pineapple

Dates

Raisins

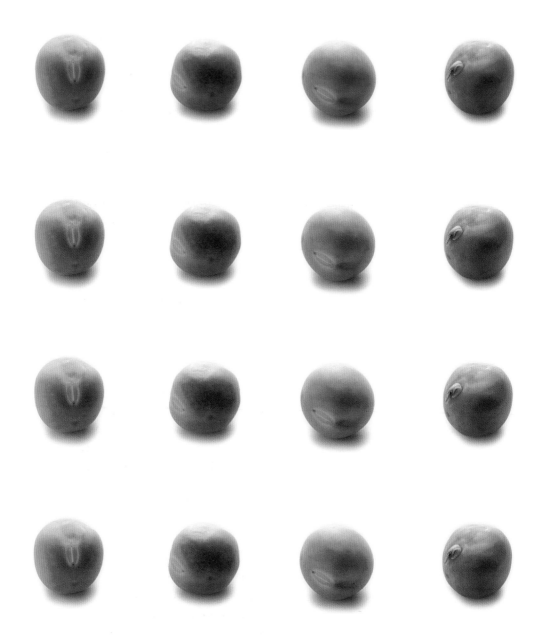

Switching to pure foods

I mentioned that energy production in your body is a chemical process. This natural chemical (or biochemical) system relies upon an adequate supply of natural nutrients from your food and drink. While modern, processed foods are depleted of many essential nutrients, pure, fresh, organic foods guarantee a supply of the nutrients we need for energy production. Some of the most important energy-boosting foods are those that are rich in vitamin A (such as carrots, green leafy vegetables, and mango), in the B-complex vitamins (such as green leafy vegetables, courgettes [zucchini], avocadoes, strawberries and, for B12, eggs and cheese), in vitamin C (including citrus fruits, broccoli and capiscums), and in the mineral iron (such as beans, lentils, broccoli and parsley). Boost these foods in your diet, and at the same time boost your energy. Easy!

How the plans work

Congratulations! You are about to give yourself an energy overhaul! Over the following pages are the three energy-boost plans, lasting a weekend (see pp.128–31), a week (pp.132–6) and a month (pp.137–9) respectively.

WHICH PLAN SHOULD I USE – WEEKEND, WEEK OR MONTH?

If you have had an isolated stressful week and are feeling physically, mentally and/or emotionally drained, then try the weekend energy-boost plan, just to relieve the short-term stress and give you a lift into the week ahead. However, if you have suffered or are suffering an extended period of stress or of illness, you would do well to dedicate a longer period of time to the plan. Aim for the week and, if you can, progress to the month. Giving yourself plenty of time for recovery will ensure that you return to the world fit, well and ready to go.

HOW ARE THE PLANS LAID OUT?

Each plan has three steps to guide you. The first step will show you how to prepare for the energy-boost – making sure that you have done all you can to have some dedicated "me" time. The second gives detailed advice on the meals you will need to eat during the plan and refers to the recipes on pages 140–53. The third step offers advice on breathing, relaxing and stretching, including an energizing meditation and foot massage.

INTRODUCING THE ENERGY-BOOST PLANS

The aim of the energy-boost plans is to return you to a state of vibrant energy by increasing your intake of foods that supply the nutrients you need to manufacture and distribute energy through your body, and by removing all the foods that sap your energy.

What to expect from the plans

If you are very tired when you begin the plans, and your lifestyle is such that you have little time to look after yourself properly, the results will amaze you. Your body will react quickly to even small changes. You may find that you sleep a lot at first. In the case of the weekend plan, this might mean that all you do is eat, meditate, stretch and rest. Listen to your body and do as it tells you.

In the long-term you will benefit from sustained, consistent energy, rather than peaks and troughs. You will sleep better, because you will not be overtired. You will develop an awareness of how you lose energy (through such things as a poor diet and lack of exercise, and stress and dehydration) and prevent them from happening. Expending energy properly and resting fully will benefit your immune system, and you may suffer fewer minor ailments, such as colds.

General rules for the energy plans

MAKE TIME FOR YOURSELF Cancel all unnecessary appointments and say no to any non-critical demands on your time and energy. This is your chance to take a step back and focus on you and your needs. Decide to relax. Make the decision not to involve yourself too much in the goings on around you – create a bubble around yourself and do all you can not to pop it.

AVOID CAFFEINE Stay away from coffee and tea as the high from caffeine is a false one. Drink lots of Max's restorative herbal tea (see p.129) instead. Drink at least 2 litres (4 pints) of pure water a day, too.

ALWAYS EAT BREAKFAST Breakfast is the most important meal of the day. A wholesome, pure-foods breakfast will help you to avoid the mid-morning energy dip that sends many of us reaching for the cookies for a quick fix.

SNACK ON PURE FOODS If, despite eating a good breakfast and hearty lunch, you have energy dips at around 11am and 3pm, don't reach for the high-GI snacks (see p.121) – have a good-GI snack instead. Try hummus and vegetable crudités (asparagus, broccoli, celery, cucumber, radish, string beans and (bell) peppers are all good-GI veggies); a low-GI fruit (see p.121) and ground nuts purée (mix a few of the fruits together, purée them, then stir in the nuts); or a heaped teaspoon of ground nuts (a mix of almonds, Brazils, walnuts and pine nuts tastes great) spooned into a serving of plain, live yogurt.

FINISH DIGESTING BEFORE YOU SLEEP Digestion is an energy-sapping activity for the body. Eat before 8pm so that your body has finished digesting by the time you go to bed, and don't drink with you meals as this dilutes the digestive juices and so increases the time digestion takes.

MIX PROTEIN AND CARBS ONLY AT LUNCHTIME When it comes to stabilizing energy, food combining in the evening is a must. If the food you eat is hard to digest, you may end up lying in bed digesting and not resting (see pp.86–7). The basic concept is not to combine carbohydrates and protein at your evening meal. An example of a bad combination is pasta (carbohydrate) and a meat (protein) sauce. A good combination would be salad or vegetables (which, other than potato, are "neutral" and so fine to eat with either protein or carbohydrate) and a piece of fresh fish (protein). However, by all means eat both carbs and protein at lunchtime as this will keep your blood sugars stable for longer, giving you a sustained energy release throughout the afternoon. As a guide to help you plan your evening meals, the following are lists of strong proteins and strong carbohydrates. In the evening you can eat foods from one list or the other, but not from both.

- Strong proteins are fish, tofu, chicken, beans (such as kidney beans or lentils), all red meats, pork, turkey and eggs.
- Strong carbohydrates are pasta, bread, potato, millet, corn, rice and quinoa.

Side-effects of the energy plans

As with the other plans in the book, the energy plans are essentially clearing your body of its old, worn-out ways. For this reason you may experience any of the following side-effects during the plans: occasional diarrhea, runny nose, occasional nausea, occasional mild sore throat, headaches, some bad breath, or a low fever. None of these is a sign that you have a cold or flu, or anything more serious. They are merely "healing crises" – signals that your body is cleaning out. In most cases the crises will be over in a day or two.

What's on the menu?

Everything that you eat over the course of the energy plans will help to stabilize your energy output. All the foods are medium- or low-GI, and many of them have additional properties that will benefit your energy levels. An oat-rich breakfast on the first day will help to soothe away the stress of the last week, as well as provide tryptophan to elevate your mood, and soluble fibre to aid your digestion. Bananas are packed with energy-making B-vitamins and potassium, while grapes contain chromium, which helps to regulate

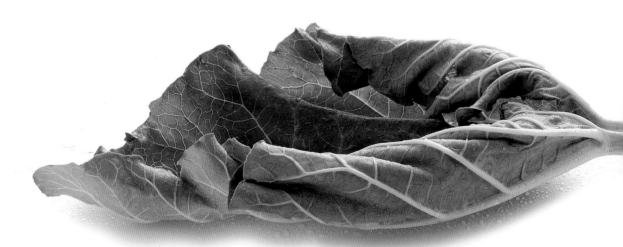

blood-sugar levels. Blueberries and mushrooms will help to support your immunity, freeing up energy for the fun things in life, and they also contain vitamin B2, which helps to convert food into energy. Eggs for breakfast will provide essential protein and iron, while salmon is rich in essential fatty acids, which will help to boost your mental energy. Best of all, desserts aren't off the menu! These low-GI, nutrient-rich puds are energy-friendly and delicious. Finally, I've suggested that before bed you drink a cup of my restorative herbal tea. The herbs in this brew both strengthen and soothe, to boost vitality during the day and also prepare you for a deep sleep at night.

The power nutrient supplements

- Chromium polynicotinate helps in the metabolism of glucose for energy and, through its action on insulin, is essential for maintaining stable blood sugars. Take between 200mcg and 400mcg a day.
- The B-complex vitamins are essential to the health of the nervous system and for proper brain function, but B5 is particularly important for adrenal function and for the correct metabolism of carbohydrates. It is always best to take all of the B-vitamins as a complex (follow the dosage on the bottle) in order not to hamper the absorption of any one of them. You can then add more B5 (100mg a day) if you are experiencing adrenal exhaustion.
- Magnesium acts as a catalyst for energy production. The dosage is between 200mg and 400mg a day.
- Siberian ginseng is an adaptogen – it helps the body to adapt to stressful situations. One of its constituents, the eleutherosides, acts on the adrenal glands, helping to prevent adrenal exhaustion. Take ginseng (according to the manufacturer's instructions) as a tea, capsule or ideally fresh plant tincture.

INTRODUCING THE WEEKEND ENERGY-BOOST PLAN

The weekend energy-boost plan covers two days and is ideal as a quick energizer at the end of a difficult week (or month, or year!), or as a way to prepare yourself for a particularly busy week ahead.

What can I achieve in a weekend?

This quick, easy-to-follow plan is a brief but powerful respite from the demands on your energy and will set you on the path to overall greater vitality. The weekend will raise your awareness so that you can carry its principles beyond the two days: you will be clear about how some foods boost energy while others sap it; you will be inspired to pay more attention to your physical needs, understanding that simple stretching and proper breathing have a role to play in keeping your energy levels up. You will end the weekend feeling more energized and getting better sleep than you have done in a long while.

How will I feel during the plan?

Don't be surprised if you don't feel full of beans after the first morning of the plan! The weekend energy-boost plan is also partly a physical detox, with fresh foods and no stimulants. If you are a big coffee- or tea-drinker you might experience caffeine withdrawal headaches. Drink plenty of water and Max's restorative herbal tea (see opposite) to keep yourself hydrated. Taking time out of your busy life can also be an emotional experience. Don't be surprised if you gain some insight into your life and relationships, some of which can cause a degree of emotional pain. If you feel emotional and vulnerable, have a feel-good warm bath or shower with your favourite essential oils (see p.130).

Finishing the energy-boost plans

Whichever energy plan you go for (weekend, week or four-week), finish on Monday morning, not on Sunday night. That morning do five minutes of stretching and deep breathing and have a quick foot massage before you begin the day. What a start to the new week! Try to remain relaxed, focused and energized no matter what the day, week, or month throws at you. When the going gets tough smile (inwardly if you have to) and take a deep, calming breath. Say the word "calm" over to yourself until you feel any stress passing.

When you finish the weekend plan, try to keep going with the "general rules" (such as eating before eight, and food combining in the evening; see p.125) for a little while longer, even making some of them habit. When you get to the end of the longer plans, don't rush back to the foods that you craved a short energy-boost ago – stick with the new dietary habits, including more low-GI foods, less caffeine and more water. You will be shocked at how quickly you will come crashing down to low-energy earth if you go back to eating and living like you did. Finally, plan to do a regular top-up plan (the weekend plan is ideal for this) every three months or so.

At the end of each plan, do something that you have wanted to do but put off because you have been too tired to do it. A visit to an art gallery? Or a day out walking with friends? Perhaps even a day at a theme park with your kids. Spoil yourself – you have the energy to have fun!

MAX'S RESTORATIVE HERBAL TEA

1 part chamomile flowers
1 part ginkgo biloba
¼ part spearmint leaves
1 part lemon balm
¼ part rose petals
⅛ part cinnamon bark
¼ part Siberian ginseng (finely chopped and ground)

Mix up a quantity of the dried tea mixture and store it in a sealed container. Use 1 tbsp per cup of tea. Leave the herbs to soak in boiling water for 5 minutes, then strain and drink. You can make up a pot and reheat the tea as you need it. If you are not partial to cinnamon, just leave it out or reduce the amount you use.

THE WEEKEND ENERGY-BOOST PLAN

Step 1: preparation

Fabulous! A weekend to yourself. If you live alone, shut the door, lose the TV remote control, cancel everything, say NO, turn off the telephone, and go into energy hibernation. You have nothing to give anyone else. Your Friday has entered the selfish zone. It's all about "me and my energy". If you live with other people, negotiate some time to yourself. Tell your partner, children, flatmates and friends that you will emerge a much more active and willing participant in their lives if they can give you this time – they will understand if you beg nicely!

Run a deep bath, get that book or magazine you really want to read and dive into the "me" zone. Use a few drops of an essential oil. Don't overdo it as you don't want stimulation from the oil, just a gentle background smell to take your mind off last week – one or two drops should be enough. Choose an essential oil you like. Some of the most relaxing are ylang ylang, rose, sandalwood and lavender (make sure you dilute the oil according to the bottle instructions and check suitability if you are pregnant or unwell). Lie back and tell the world to back off. If you don't have a bath or don't like to soak, have a shower, and scrub yourself down with a natural shower gel. Go to bed early and do the meditation, opposite. On Saturday night opt for an early night after a gentle walk. What utter luxury you selfish being!

Step 2: menu plan

DAY ONE

Energy:aid juice Carrot mania (p.142)

Breakfast Aztec porridge (p.140)

Lunch Green goddess salad (p.146)

Dinner Wild mushroom and brown rice risotto (p.150), followed by Blueberries with lashings of banana sauce (p.152) for dessert

Before bed Max's restorative herbal tea (p.129)

DAY TWO

Energy:aid smoothie Marrakech express (p.145)

Breakfast Scrambled and easy (p.140)

Lunch Steamed salmon with miso (p.148)

Dinner Warm chicken and blueberry salad with lime dressing (p.149), followed by Creamy rice pudding (p.152) for dessert

Before bed Max's restorative herbal tea (p.129)

SNACKS

Eating low-GI, pure foods little and often will help to regulate your energy levels and give you a sustained energy output, so snacks are definitely not banned from this weekend plan. However, avoid sugary snacks, such as cookies and chocolate, which will send your blood-sugar levels yo-yoing, and instead opt for the hummus and crudités, puréed fruit, or mixed nut and yogurt options I suggest on page 125.

Step 3: action

Aim to do 15 to 20 minutes of Breathing, Relaxing, Stretching (BRS) each day during the energy-boost plan. You can use the stretches in Chapter 6 too.

BREATHING   Correct breathing draws oxygen deep into the lungs, energizing you at a deep level. Shallow or incomplete breathing leads to tiredness and low mental energy. Practise full, energizing breathing each morning. Stand in front of an open window and inhale deeply for a few minutes. Breathe right into the abdomen. Do not hyperventilate or you may fall over!

RELAXING   It seems like a contradiction to say that relaxation energizes you, but releasing your mind from all its little worries and letting go subtle muscle tensions in the body frees up a lot of energy for you to use constructively in your day. Try a meditation (see right). Meditation is not about stopping your thoughts and sitting in silence, but about watching your thoughts without getting involved in them. Have a go – nothing ventured, nothing gained!

STRETCHING   Stretching releases muscles, improves blood-flow and increases the amount of energizing oxygen in your tissues. Try this stretch when you wake up: stand tall, with your feet wide apart. Inhale and raise your arms, elbows straight, wrists limply bent. Exhale as you swing your trunk downward from the waist. Allow your arms and head to swing in and out of the space between your legs. Relax as you swing back and forth. Inhale as you stand tall. Repeat five times.

SO–HUM MEDITATION

1   Loosen any tight clothing and sit comfortably in a position that you can hold without fidgeting – say cross-legged on the floor, or in a chair with your feet firmly on the ground. Close your eyes. Breathe in and out gently, relaxing all of your muscles as you do so.

2   Now turn your full focus to your breathing. Listen to the sound that your breath makes as it enters and exits your body. The sound as it enters is "SO". The sound as it exits is "HUM".

3   Imagine the sound in your mind. SO–HUM. SO–HUM. A gentle and regular rhythm and sound.

4   Try to let the sound of the breath fill your awareness. Really focus on the "SO" and the "HUM".

5   If your mind wanders and you start to think about other things, gently bring your awareness back to your breath. Practise this for anything up to 30 minutes on both days.

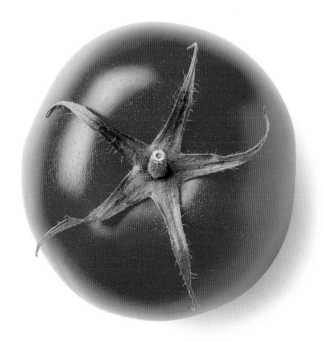

THE DEEPER ENERGY-BOOSTS

You've successfully completed the weekend energy-boost plan – congratulations! Now the one- and four-week energy-boost plans await you. Use them to restore a deep-rooted sense of vitality that will help you to enjoy every minute of life to the full.

Why should I choose a longer plan?

Simple. Because no-one can have too much energy! The weekend is a brilliant way to start and an excellent pick-me-up after an especially hard week, but a weekend is not really long enough to address adrenal exhaustion (see p.119). Another five days of energy detox should really help to rest your adrenal glands and get them back into shape, and will give the energy nutrients (most importantly the B-vitamins and magnesium, which are so important for energy production; and chromium, which helps to regulate blood-sugar levels) in pure foods extra time to take effect. A full four weeks will completely overhaul your adrenal glands and restore the overall effectiveness of your otherwise tired and depleted nervous system.

How can I juggle the longer plans with my everyday routine?

We said at the beginning of the weekend energy-boost plan that you were entering the "selfish zone". While being in this zone is going to be fairly easy over a weekend, unless you can take a whole week or month out of your normal routine, it is going to prove more difficult and impractical over the longer plans. However, now is the time for some assertiveness training – you will be amazed by how liberating (and energizing) you find it to stand up for your right to more time for yourself, even when you remain sensitive to the rights and needs of others. Be honest about your feelings and your needs. Learn to prioritize. If something can wait, let it wait. Be bold and ask for help to ease your load, even if it is for only these few weeks. Ask someone else to do the school run, or to drop the kids at soccer or ballet, or to walk the dog. If you are at work, reschedule any non-urgent meetings for after your energy-boost (you will be better equipped to deal with them then anyway) and mark out a specific time each day – 30 minutes, or an hour at most – for solving other people's problems. Politely let your team and colleagues know in advance when you are available to help them so that they don't make constant demands on your time and energy. Finally, before agreeing to do anything, ask yourself "Am I the right person for this job?" Be convinced before you answer yes, and don't be afraid to say no (nicely, but firmly) to those who make unnecessary or inappropriate demands on you.

Celebrate your new energy

Plan a weekend away. We all need something to look forward to, and while I'm convinced that after an energy-boost plan you will never want to go back to the old diet, old routines and old you, a little motivational goal never did anyone any harm. As far as energy is concerned, regular get-aways break up a busy life into manageable chunks – it's easier to face a difficult week if you know at the end of it you have something lovely to do. A short break to a city you have always wanted to visit, a camping trip with your family, a visit to distant friends, or a few days in the hills or mountains are all superb ways to congratulate yourself on completing an energy-boost.

MAX'S MOTIVATOR

NEVER WORRY IF YOU HAVE A WOBBLY MOMENT DURING THE PLAN

If ever you feel that you are about to stray from the plan, or if you have actually slipped up, don't be hard on yourself. Have a cup of Max's restorative herbal tea, pick yourself up and get back on the energy-boost. Don't think in terms of success and failure. Remember that every little bit you do do, every minute you spend eating well and every breathing or stretching session you undertake, does you good.

THE ONE-WEEK ENERGY-BOOST PLAN

Step 1: preparation

The kindest way to prepare yourself for the one-week plan is to adopt some time-management strategies. As well as the assertiveness advice on pages 132–3, all of the following will make life easier on you, freeing up your time to concentrate on getting back your vitality.

- Make daily and weekly written lists of things that you need to do. Get the list out of your head and onto paper so that you don't have to take up precious mind power with a mental diary. A written list will also help you to put tasks into clear order of priority. Put the most urgent things at the top and work down in descending order of importance. If you don't get to the items at the bottom on one day, it doesn't matter – put them at the top of the following day's list.
- Handle household or office paperwork only once – read it; then answer it, throw it out or delegate it. However, don't postpone important matters that are unpleasant. Procrastination will not make things better, it will just play on your mind, sapping that mental energy.
- Set aside a regular time for phone calls – better to do them in one burst and have them out of the way. And as for those endless emails – again, schedule some dedicated time for them, and stick to it. Only rarely will there be something that can't wait until first thing tomorrow.

Step 2: menu plan

A quick reminder: never skip breakfast! A solid morning meal gets the body making energy efficiently right from the beginning of the day. Stress-relieving oats, in the form of porridge and muesli, will help mobilize your energy with their high B-vitamin content, as will millet (in The quick cheat), which is higher in magnesium than any other cereal. This week's lunches include delicious buckwheat pancakes. Buckwheat, a member of the grass family, is packed with protein to provide energy and is a fantastic grain to help control blood sugars. (It is also very high in bone-building calcium.) Avocado (in the Green goddess salad) is one of nature's wonderfoods and great for your energy. It is packed with B-vitamins, which help to reduce stress, convert food to energy, and maintain a healthy nervous system; and also contains heaps of fibre to keep your digestion working at its best, and essential fatty acids to boost your brain power. All of the meals are low- or medium-GI, of course, to try to balance out those energy highs and lows. If you need to snack, see my energy-friendly options on page 125, or even have an energy-boost smoothie (see pp.144–5).

NOTE: In the following menu plan, use days one and two from the weekend energy-boost. Turn to page 136 for Step 3: action for the one-week plan.

THE ONE-WEEK MENU PLAN

DAY 3

Energy:aid juice Blast of purple (p.142)

Breakfast Proper Swiss muesli (p.141)

Lunch Moroccan harira soup (p.146)

Dinner Stir-fried sesame chicken (p.149), followed by Silken fruit delight (p.153) for dessert

Before bed Max's restorative herbal tea (p.129)

DAY 4

Energy:aid smoothie Summer sunshine (p.144)

Breakfast The quick cheat (p.141)

Lunch Spinach and orange salad with Brazil nut dukka (p.148)

Dinner Bag-baked hoki with spicy tomatoes and steamed green beans (p.150), followed by Macro fruit purée (p.153)

Before bed Max's restorative herbal tea (p.129)

DAY 5

Energy:aid juice Tricolour (p.143)

Breakfast Proper Swiss muesli (p.141)

Lunch Steamed salmon with miso (p.148)

Dinner Wild mushroom and brown rice risotto (p.150), followed by Creamy rice pudding for dessert (p.152)

Before bed Max's restorative herbal tea (p.129)

DAY 6

Energy:aid smoothie Tropical punch (p.144)

Breakfast Scrambled and easy (p.140)

Lunch Buckwheat crespolini (p.147)

Dinner Warm chicken and blueberry salad with lime dressing (p.149), followed by Creamy rice pudding (p.152) for dessert

Before bed Max's restorative herbal tea (p.129)

DAY 7

Energy:aid juice Vive la France (p.143)

Breakfast Aztec porridge (p.140)

Lunch Green goddess salad (p.146)

Dinner Mixed vegetable curry (p.151), followed by Blueberries with lashings of banana sauce (p.152) for dessert

Before bed Max's restorative herbal tea (p.129)

SNACKS

As with the weekend detox, snack on low-GI, pure foods little and often to help to regulate your energy levels and give you a sustained energy output. However, avoid any sugary snacks, such as cookies and chocolate, which will cause your blood-sugar levels to yo-yo, and instead opt for the hummus and crudités, puréed fruit, or mixed nut and yogurt options I suggest on page 125.

Step 3: action

BREATHING, RELAXING, STRETCHING (BRS)
It's essential for your energy that you practise BRS every day. By now you should be familiar with the BRS advice in the weekend plan – keep up the good work throughout the week; or if you fancy a change, use some of the additional advice given in Chapter 6. In particular you should be settling into the idea of a daily meditation. Either that or you are about to give up because it's so hard to get your mind to take a back seat. Please don't give up. Meditation does take practice and if you are finding it hard, just try to sit still and listen intently to a piece of favourite music or to birdsong. Try to empty your mind of everything but the sound. Once you can do this happily, go back to the exercise on page 131 and try again. Finally, don't forget to exercise (see pp.214–17) – using energy, makes energy!

SLEEPING
Although we might think that the more sleep we get, the more energy we will have, often the opposite is true. Too much sleep can lead to feelings of physical, mental and emotional fatigue, and even depression. Aim for eight hours a night throughout the plan, say from 11pm to 7am.

FOOT MASSAGE
Kick start your energy-boost day with an energizing reflexology foot massage (see right). This doesn't need to be complicated – just a nice rub of the souls of your feet, focusing on the adrenal, head and liver points. The pressure on these points will help to restore balance in your energy regulators. You can use either massage oil or cream. I prefer natural grape seed oil or apricot kernel oil.

ENERGIZING FOOT MASSAGE

1 In this foot massage you will use reflexology (zone therapy) points to stimulate your body's energy. Before you begin, pinpoint the liver, adrenal and head points on each foot (see diagram, below).

2 Rub some massage oil into your hands to lubricate them and to warm the oil. Don't use too much oil as this will make your hands and feet too slippery and you will not be able to work the points properly.

3 Start on your right foot. Grasp it gently, using your right hand to hold the top of your foot, and rest it lightly on your left knee. Turn the foot gently so that its sole faces you. Using the thumb of your left hand, rub the sole, the heel and the toes all over. Use firm pressure, but don't press so hard that it hurts.

4 Focus now on the adrenal, head and liver points. Play around, using your thumb and fingers, knuckles and fists to massage in turn the three points. Apply enough pressure so that you feel a small amount of pain at first, which will ease as you work each part of the foot. Take your time, gently exploring tender areas. When you are ready, swap your feet over to massage the left foot, resting it on your right knee.

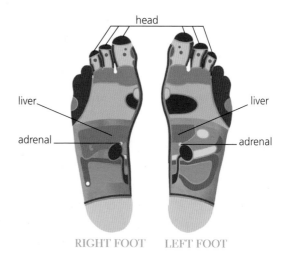

RIGHT FOOT   LEFT FOOT

EXTENDING THE PLAN TO FOUR WEEKS

Four weeks of energy-boosting will really sort out your adrenal function and give you the chance to approach life with a renewed outlook. You will feel fresh, positive and full of vitality; the tired lines on your face will have disappeared and your eyes will sparkle.

Preparing, eating and BRS

Each week and then each day, continue to make lists of the tasks you need to complete, as well as keeping up with the other assertiveness and time-management techniques (see pp.132–3 and 134). In addition to the breathing, relaxing and stretching routines you already know, try to spend at least 15 minutes each day in dedicated deep breathing to bring oxygen, and so energy, into your lungs. Any of the exercises on pages 222–3 will do. The four-week menu plan is on pages 138–9, but if you feel like turbo-charging your energy, and you are otherwise fit and well, swap one of the menu days for a one-day juice fast. Instead of meals, drink five fresh juices during the day. Use each of the four recipes on pages 142–3, and then repeat one.

Exercise

I can't stress how important exercise is for energy-making. If you are new to exercise, consider walking for half an hour each day. Try to get your heart rate up to around 120 beats per minute in the half-hour. This will improve your circulation and flood the organs and muscles with oxygenated, energizing blood, leaving you feeling calm but full of vitality. Aim to be doing an hour of walking or other exercise every day by the end of the four weeks.

THE FOUR-WEEK ENERGY-BOOST MENU PLAN

Use the menu plans from the weekend and week energy-boosts for your first week; here are the menu plans for weeks two to four. Begin each day with a juice or smoothie (see pp.142–5) and end each day with Max's restorative herbal tea (see p.129). Rules on snacks apply as they did for the shorter energy-boost plans: steer clear of the sugar – no cookies or chocolate – and try my suggestions on page 125 instead; or have another smoothie. Feel free to juggle the recipes according to your preference, but try to keep the variety so that you benefit fully from the whole range of energy-giving nutrients.

WEEK TWO

DAY	BREAKFAST	LUNCH	DINNER
Monday	Aztec porridge (p.140)	Green goddess salad (p.146)	Bag-baked hoki with spicy tomatoes and steamed green beans (p.150)
Tuesday	Scrambled and easy (p.140)	Moroccan harira soup (p.146)	Mixed vegetable curry (p.151)
Wednesday	Proper Swiss muesli (p.141)	Spinach and orange salad with Brazil nut dukka (p.148)	Wild mushroom and brown rice risotto (p.150)
Thursday	The quick cheat (p.141)	Green goddess salad (p.146)	Stir-fried sesame chicken (p.149)
Friday	Aztec porridge (p.140)	Buckwheat crespolini (p.147)	Bag-baked hoki with spicy tomatoes and steamed green beans (p.150)
Saturday	Scrambled and easy (p.140)	Steamed salmon with miso (p.148)	Wild mushroom and brown rice risotto (p.150)
Sunday	The quick cheat (p.141)	Moroccan harira soup (p.146)	Warm chicken and blueberry salad with lime dressing (p.149)

WEEK THREE

DAY	BREAKFAST	LUNCH	DINNER
Monday	Aztec porridge (p.140)	Buckwheat crespolini (p.147)	Mixed vegetable curry (p.151)
Tuesday	Scrambled and easy (p.140)	Spinach and orange salad with Brazil nut dukka (p.148)	Bag-baked hoki with spicy tomatoes and steamed green beans (p.150)
Wednesday	Proper Swiss muesli (p.141)	Moroccan harira soup (p.146)	Stir-fried sesame chicken (p.149)
Thursday	The quick cheat (p.141)	Green goddess salad (p.146)	Mixed vegetable curry (p.151)
Friday	Aztec porridge (p.140)	Steamed salmon with miso (p.148)	Warm chicken and blueberry salad with lime dressing (p.149)
Saturday	Scrambled and easy (p.140)	Spinach and orange salad with Brazil nut dukka (p.148)	Wild mushroom and brown rice risotto (p.150)
Sunday	Proper Swiss muesli (p.141)	Buckwheat crespolini (p.147)	Bag-baked hoki with spicy tomatoes and steamed green beans (p.150)

WEEK FOUR

DAY	BREAKFAST	LUNCH	DINNER
Monday	The quick cheat (p.141)	Moroccan harira soup (p.146)	Warm chicken and blueberry salad with lime dressing (p.149)
Tuesday	Aztec porridge (p.140)	Green goddess salad (p.146)	Wild mushroom and brown rice risotto (p.150)
Wednesday	Scrambled and easy (p.140)	Steamed salmon with miso (p.148)	Bag-baked hoki with spicy tomatoes and steamed green beans (p.150)
Thursday	Proper Swiss muesli (p.141)	Spinach and orange salad with Brazil nut dukka (p.148)	Mixed vegetable curry (p.151)
Friday	The quick cheat (p.141)	Buckwheat crespolini (p.147)	Stir-fried sesame chicken (p.149)
Saturday	Aztec porridge (p.140)	Steamed salmon with miso (p.148)	Wild mushroom and brown rice risotto (p.150)
Sunday	Scrambled and easy (p.140)	Moroccan harira soup (p.146)	Bag-baked hoki with spicy tomatoes and steamed green beans (p.150)

ENERGY BREAKFASTS

Aztec porridge

SERVES 1
PREPARATION TIME 5 MINUTES
COOKING TIME 5 MINUTES

Soya (soy), goat's or rice milk (for soaking)
Handful (25g/1oz/⅛ cup) rolled organic quinoa
Handful (25g/1oz/⅛ cup) rolled organic oats
10 blueberries or raspberries, crushed
1 small pear (or any seasonal soft fruit), chopped
1 tbsp live culture yogurt

1 Cover the grains in soya, goat's or rice milk and soak overnight.

2 In the morning add a little water so that you cover the grains again, and then cook the grains for 5 minutes or until they are soft.

3 Serve hot with crushed berries, chopped pear and a dollop of fresh, live yogurt.

Scrambled and easy

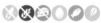

SERVES 1
PREPARATION TIME 2 MINUTES
COOKING TIME 4 MINUTES

1 tbsp extra virgin olive oil
40g/1½oz organic smoked salmon, chopped
1 tsp chopped shallots (scallions)
2 medium organic, free-range eggs
Pinch chopped parsley

1 Drizzle a little olive oil into a small, heated, non-stick frying pan (skillet). Add the chopped salmon and chopped shallots (scallions). Stir for 1 minute on a medium heat.

2 Crack the eggs into the mixture. Keep stirring with a wooden spoon until the eggs are light and fluffy.

3 Sprinkle over the parsley and serve immediately.

Proper Swiss muesli

SERVES 1
PREPARATION TIME 5 MINUTES

Milk for soaking (use any milk, unless you are allergic or sensitive to cow's milk – in which case use goat's, sheep's or soya/soy milk)

Handful (25g/1oz/⅛ cup) rolled organic oats

Handful (25g/1oz/⅛ cup) rolled organic millet

Handful (25g/1oz/⅛ cup) rolled organic rye

1 tsp organic raisins

1 small apple, washed and chopped

1 tbsp berries (blueberries, raspberries, strawberries and/or bilberries)

2 tbsp live culture yogurt

1 Soak the grains overnight in the milk and soak the raisins overnight in water. (If you do not like raisins you may use fresh grapes, sliced in half.)

2 In a bowl mix together the grains, raisins, chopped apple and berries. Serve at room temperature with the yogurt.

The quick cheat

SERVES 1
PREPARATION TIME 4 MINUTES

Handful (55g/2oz/¼ cup) puffed brown rice (available from most health food stores and leading supermarkets)

Handful (55g/2oz/¼ cup) puffed millet

Handful (55g/2oz/¼ cup) puffed corn

Soya (soy), goat's or sheep's milk to taste

1 tsp almonds and hazelnuts, ground

1 banana or pear, thinly sliced

1 Add equal amounts of the puffed grains to a bowl and add the milk.

2 Sprinkle the nuts over the cereal and add the fruit.

ENERGY JUICES

Carrot mania

SERVES 1
PREPARATION TIME 5 MINUTES

3 apples
6 carrots
2.5cm/1in ginger, roughly chopped (optional)

1   Wash the apples thoroughly in warm water to
    remove the wax layer (sometimes added to preserve
    shelf life) and scrub the carrots.

2   Juice all the ingredients together, pour into a glass
    and serve.

Blast of purple

SERVES 1
PREPARATION TIME 5 MINUTES

55g/2oz/¼ cup blueberries
2 apples
1 grapefruit, peeled
2.5cm/1in fresh ginger, roughly chopped (optional)
1 tsp raw honey (optional – preferably without!)

Juice all of the ingredients together in a juicer
and serve in a tall glass.

Vive la France

SERVES 1
PREPARATION TIME 5 MINUTES

5cm/2in ginger root (or to taste), peeled
1 lemon, peeled
1 large bunch red grapes (preferably seedless)
Distilled water

Juice all the ingredients except the water together.
Dilute with the water as necessary and serve.

Tricolour

SERVES 1
PREPARATION TIME 4 MINUTES

6 strawberries
2 kiwis
1 orange

1   Wash the strawberries thoroughly and peel the
    orange and kiwi.

2   Juice all the ingredients together and serve.

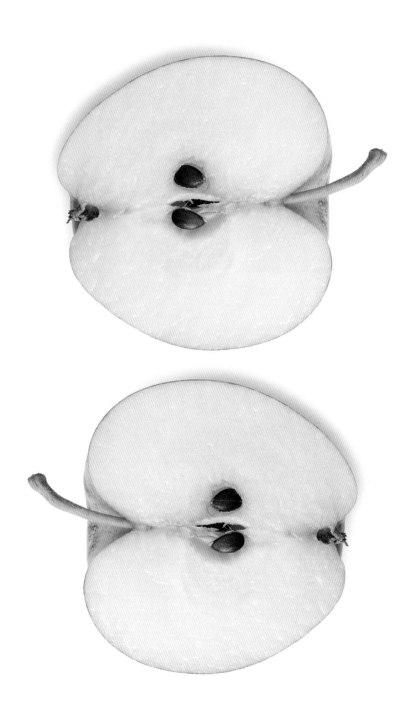

ENERGY SMOOTHIES

Summer sunshine

SERVES 1
PREPARATION TIME 5 MINUTES

225ml/8 fl oz/1 cup fresh orange juice
15 strawberries
2 medium or 1 large banana
2 tbsp linseed (flax seed) meal (available from health food stores or make your own by grinding the organic linseeds [flax seeds] in a coffee grinder)

Place all the ingredients together in a blender and blend until creamy. Pour into a glass and serve immediately.

Tropical punch

SERVES 1
PREPARATION TIME 8 MINUTES

1 green coconut with plenty of juice
1 large, very ripe banana
2 thick slices of pineapple, chopped

1 Crack open the coconut, or chop a hole in it. Empty all the liquid from the coconut into a blender (not a juicer).

2 Add the banana and chopped pineapple and blend. Pour into a glass and serve immediately.

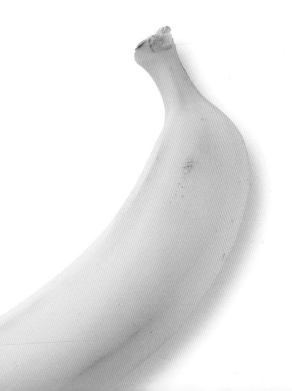

Marrakech express

SERVES 1
PREPARATION TIME 5 MINUTES

1 small, ripe papaya, skinned and de-seeded
55g/2oz/¼ cup blueberries or raspberries
1 ripe banana
2 fresh dates, de-stoned and chopped
110ml/4 fl oz/½ cup soya (soy) or rice milk to dilute
Cinnamon to taste (optional)

Place all the ingredients in a blender and blend until smooth. Pour into a glass and serve immediately.

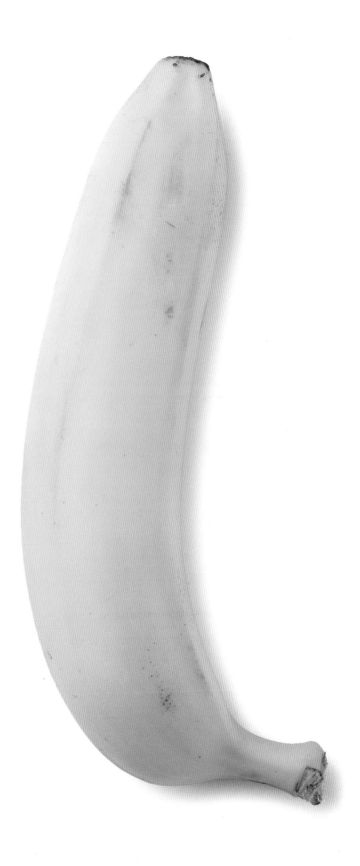

ENERGY LUNCHES

Green goddess salad

SERVES 2
PREPARATION TIME 20 MINUTES
COOKING TIME 15 MINUTES

85g/3oz/⅓ cup quinoa, rinsed
160ml/5 fl oz/⅔ cup water
1 large avocado, peeled, stoned and sliced
¼ cucumber, halved and sliced
6 salad onions, trimmed and finely sliced
2 large handfuls alfalfa sprouts, or similar sprouted seeds such as cress
Small bunch coriander (cilantro)
2 tbsp fresh lemon juice
2 tsp extra virgin olive oil
1 medium tomato, sliced

1 Cook the quinoa according to the packet instructions. When cooked, spread the quinoa out on a plate and leave to cool for 10 minutes.

2 Put the cooled quinoa, avocado, cucumber, salad onions, alfalfa sprouts and coriander (cilantro) leaves into a large bowl and toss with the lemon juice. Transfer to plates and drizzle over the olive oil. Top with the tomato slices.

Moroccan harira soup

SERVES 2
PREPARATION TIME 10 MINUTES (PLUS SOAKING)
COOKING TIME 1 HOUR 40 MINUTES

2 tbsp chickpeas (garbanzos), soaked
4 tbsp pearl barley, rinsed
1 small onion, peeled and coarsely chopped
1 large stick celery, cut into 5mm/¼in slices
1 medium carrot, peeled and cut into 5mm/¼in cubes
½ tsp ground cinnamon
½ tsp turmeric
1 tsp fresh ginger, grated
1 tbsp extra virgin olive oil
750ml/25 fl oz/3⅛ cups vegetable stock
1 x 110g/4oz skinless chicken breast, in 1cm/½in cubes
¼ medium red chilli, deseeded and diced, to serve
Small bunch coriander (cilantro), to serve
2 lemon quarters, to serve

1 Put the drained chickpeas (garbanzos) and pearl barley in a saucepan. Cover with cold water. Place over a high heat and boil rapidly for 10 minutes. Meanwhile, put the onion, celery, carrot, spices and ginger in a large pan with the olive oil and cook over a low heat for 8 minutes.

2 Drain the barley and chickpeas (garbanzos) and add to the vegetables, with the stock. Cover the pan and simmer for 1 hour 20 minutes. You can add water if the soup looks too thick. Add the chicken and cook for a further 10 minutes.

3 Ladle the soup into bowls, sprinkle over the chilli and coriander (cilantro) leaves and serve with lemon quarters to squeeze into the soup.

Buckwheat crespolini

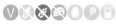

SERVES 2
PREPARATION TIME 1 HOUR AND 10 MINUTES
COOKING TIME 20 MINUTES

Pancakes
55g/2oz/¼ cup buckwheat
1 large organic, free-range egg
150ml/5 fl oz/⅔ cup soya (soy) milk
3–4 gratings nutmeg
1 tbsp organic sunflower oil, for frying

Sauce
1 shallot (scallion), peeled and finely chopped
1 tbsp extra virgin olive oil
1 small clove garlic, peeled and crushed

450g/1lb/2 cups ripe tomatoes, seeded and roughly chopped
3 tbsp water
2 tsp lemon juice
Large bunch fresh basil (reserve 12 small leaves to serve)
Small bunch fresh oregano

Filling
1 tbsp extra virgin olive oil
6 large handfuls fresh spinach leaves
2 tbsp pine nuts, lightly toasted
9–10 gratings of nutmeg

Topping
1 medium ball buffalo mozzarella, diced

1 To make the pancakes, sift the buckwheat flour into a bowl. Add the egg and stir in with a wooden spoon into a thick paste. Add one third of the soya (soy) milk and beat. Add the rest of the milk in two lots, beating well to make a smooth batter. Season with grated nutmeg and stand for 5 minutes.

2 Pour the oil in a 20cm/8in non-stick frying pan (skillet) and place over a medium heat until the oil is shimmering. Pour out the oil into a small heatproof bowl, leaving a thin layer on the bottom of the pan. Stir the pancake batter, then pour about 3 tbsp into the pan and swirl it around. Cook for 1 minute until browned underneath, then flip over with a spatula and cook the other side for a minute. Transfer the cooked pancake to a plate.

3 Use a piece of kitchen paper dipped in the extra oil to grease the bottom of the pan and repeat the pancake cooking process until all the batter is used up. It should make about four pancakes. Stack the pancakes on the plate when cooked.

4 To make the sauce, put the shallot (scallion) and olive oil in a pan over a low heat and cook gently

for 4 minutes, until the shallot (scallion) turns translucent. Add the garlic; cook for 1 minute. Add the tomatoes and water, simmer and cook for 10 minutes. Add the lemon juice, basil and oregano and blitz with a hand blender.

5 To make the filling, gently heat the olive oil in a large pan, add the spinach and stir until it has wilted. Tip into a colander and drain off as much liquid as possible, pressing down with the back of a spoon. Transfer to a bowl and add the pine nuts. Season with the grated nutmeg.

6 To cook the crespolini, preheat the oven to 180°C/fan 160°C/350°F/gas 4. Lay out four pancakes and divide the spinach mixture between them, piling it on one side of each pancake. Roll up the pancakes like cannelloni and lay in a small baking dish, seam side down. Spoon over the tomato sauce and scatter over the diced mozzarella.

7 Bake for 20 minutes until the mozzarella has melted and the sauce is bubbling. Scatter over the reserved basil leaves before serving.

Spinach and orange salad with Brazil nut dukka

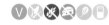

SERVES 2
PREPARATION TIME 30 MINUTES

85g/3oz/⅓ cup quinoa, rinsed thoroughly
160ml/5 fl oz/⅔ cup water
85g/3oz/⅔ cup Brazil nuts, roughly chopped
1 tsp coriander seeds, crushed
½ tsp cumin seeds, crushed
1 tbsp sesame seeds
2 large handfuls baby spinach leaves
2 large oranges, peel and pith removed and segmented
4 tbsp extra virgin olive oil
2 tbsp fresh lemon juice

1   Cook the quinoa in water following the packet instructions. When cooked, spread the quinoa out on a plate and leave to cool for 10 minutes.

2   Whilst the quinoa is cooking, make the dukka. Put the Brazil nuts in a non-stick pan and dry-fry over a low heat for 2 minutes. Add the coriander, cumin and sesame seeds and cook for another 2 minutes, stirring constantly. Transfer to a small bowl and leave to cool slightly.

3   Put the spinach, orange segments, quinoa and dukka in a large bowl. Whisk the olive oil and lemon juice together in a small bowl. Pour the dressing over the salad and toss well.

Steamed salmon with miso

SERVES 2
PREPARATION TIME 10 MINUTES
COOKING TIME 35 MINUTES

1 large sheet dried kombu (an edible kelp)
6 dried shiitake mushrooms
1 small shallot (scallion), peeled and thinly sliced
1 small knob fresh ginger (15g/½oz), thinly sliced
750ml/25 fl oz/3⅛ cups water
110g/4oz buckwheat soba noodles
2 x 110g/4oz organic salmon fillets
1 head pak choi (110g/4oz), leaves separated
2 tsp low-sodium soy sauce (optional)
Small bunch coriander (cilantro), to serve

1   To make the miso soup, put the kombu, mushrooms, shallot (scallion), ginger and water in a saucepan and place over a medium heat. Bring up to a simmer, cover and cook for 20 minutes.

2   Meanwhile, cook the noodles in plenty of boiling water for 3–4 minutes, then drain and rinse with cold water.

3   Put the salmon fillets skin side down in a steamer that fits snugly over a saucepan. Put the steamer over the saucepan and cover with the lid. Cook for 10–12 minutes until the salmon is opaque and just starting to flake. Remove the steamer and keep the salmon warm.

4   Strain the stock and reserve the mushrooms. Put the stock back in the saucepan and add the pak choi. Simmer over a medium heat for 1 minute. Slice the mushrooms and add to the stock with the noodles and soy sauce (optional). Ladle the soup into wide bowls and top with the salmon. Sprinkle over the coriander (cilantro) leaves.

ENERGY DINNERS

Stir-fried sesame chicken

SERVES 2
PREPARATION TIME 15 MINUTES
COOKING TIME 8–10 MINUTES

1 tbsp extra virgin olive oil

2 x 100g/4oz skinless organic chicken breast, cut into 5mm/¼in wide strips

½ tsp fresh ginger, grated

1 small clove garlic, peeled and crushed

1 medium head broccoli (150g/5½oz), broken into small florets

6 cobs baby corn, cut in half lengthways

1 medium carrot, cut into matchsticks

4 tbsp water

Large handful (85g/3oz) mange tout

2 tsp sesame seeds

2 tsp sesame oil

1 Put the olive oil in a wok over a high heat, add the chicken and cook for 2 minutes. Add the ginger, garlic, broccoli, corn, carrot and water and cook for a further 2 minutes. Add the mange tout and cook for 2–3 minutes, until the vegetables are just tender and the chicken is cooked through.

2 Add the sesame seeds and cook for 30 seconds, then take the wok off the heat and stir in the sesame oil before serving.

Warm chicken and blueberry salad with lime dressing

SERVES 2
PREPARATION TIME 20 MINUTES
COOKING TIME 8 MINUTES

2 x 110g/4oz organic chicken breasts, skinless and boneless

Finely grated zest of 1 organic unwaxed lime, plus 3 tbsp juice

4 tbsp extra virgin olive oil

1 cos (romaine) lettuce, outer leaves removed, torn into pieces

6 salad onions, trimmed and finely sliced

1 medium avocado, peeled, stoned and sliced

Large handful (75g/2½oz) fresh blueberries

1 Put the chicken breasts between two large pieces of greaseproof paper and use a rolling pin to flatten the breasts into escalopes around 1cm/½in thick. Put in a shallow dish and sprinkle over the lime zest, 2 tbsp olive oil and 2 tsp lime juice. Turn the chicken to coat in the marinade and leave for 10 minutes.

2 Put the lettuce, salad onions, avocado and blueberries into a large bowl. Whisk together the remaining olive oil and lime juice in a small bowl and pour over the salad. Toss to coat in the dressing.

3 Griddle or grill (broil) the chicken breasts for 3–4 minutes on each side, until cooked through. Slice into strips and scatter over the salad.

Wild mushroom and brown rice risotto

SERVES 2
PREPARATION TIME 10 MINUTES
COOKING TIME 50 MINUTES

1 small shallot (scallion), peeled and finely chopped
1 tbsp plus 1 tsp extra virgin olive oil
1 fat clove garlic, peeled and crushed
1 tsp fresh thyme leaves
225g/8oz/1 cup brown rice, rinsed
300ml/10 fl oz/1¼ cups vegetable stock
300ml/10 fl oz/1¼ cups water
4 handfuls (250g/9oz) mixed wild mushrooms, sliced
2 tbsp lemon juice
Small bunch flat leaf parsley, chopped

1 Put the shallot (scallion) and 1 tsp olive oil in a saucepan over a low heat and cook for 5 minutes.

2 Add the garlic and thyme and cook for 1 minute, then add the rice, stock and water. Turn up the heat to medium and simmer for 40 minutes, until the rice is cooked. Add a little extra water if the rice becomes too dry.

3 Stir-fry the mushrooms with 1 tbsp olive oil for 5–6 minutes in a wok or large frying pan (skillet) on a medium heat. Just before serving, stir the mushrooms into the cooked rice, with the lemon juice and parsley.

Bag-baked hoki with spicy tomatoes and steamed green beans

SERVES 2
PREPARATION TIME 15 MINUTES
COOKING TIME 10 MINUTES

2 x 110g/4oz skinless hoki fillet steaks
10 baby plum tomatoes, quartered
2 salad onions, trimmed and sliced
½ fresh red chilli, deseeded and finely chopped (for medium heat)
½ tsp fresh ginger, grated
2 tsp lemon juice
2 large handfuls (170g/6oz) fine green beans, trimmed
Small bunch coriander (cilantro), chopped, to serve

1 Preheat the oven to 200°C/fan 180°C/400°F/gas 6. Cut four rectangles of greaseproof paper measuring 43 x 38cm/17 x 15in.

2 Lay two pieces of greaseproof paper out flat and put a second piece of paper on top of each to make a double layer. Put a piece of hoki in the centre of each rectangle.

3 Put the tomatoes in a small bowl and add the salad onions, chilli, ginger and lemon juice. Mix well, then spoon evenly on top of the hoki.

4 Bring the long edges of the greaseproof paper together and fold over a couple of times to hold them together. Roll down the edges to seal and twist the corners to secure. Put on a baking sheet and cook on the top shelf for 10 minutes. While the hoki is cooking, steam the green beans for 8 minutes, until tender.

5 Remove the hoki from the oven. Put the beans on a plate then lift the hoki and tomatoes on to the beans using a fish slice. Pour over any juices and sprinkle over the coriander (cilantro).

Mixed vegetable curry

SERVES 2
PREPARATION TIME 20 MINUTES
COOKING TIME 50 MINUTES

110g/4oz/½ cup brown rice, rinsed

1 small onion, peeled and finely chopped

1 tbsp extra virgin olive oil

1 fat clove garlic, peeled and crushed

1 tsp fresh ginger, grated

½ red chilli, deseeded and chopped (for medium heat)

1 tsp ground cumin

½ tsp ground coriander

½ tsp turmeric

Large pinch cayenne pepper

450g/1lb ripe tomatoes

300ml/10 fl oz/1¼ cups water

½ medium cauliflower (140g/5oz), broken into small florets

Handful (75g/2½oz) green beans, cut into 2.5cm/1in lengths

Large handful baby spinach leaves

9–10 gratings nutmeg

Small bunch coriander (cilantro), chopped, to serve

1 Put the rice on to cook, according to the packet instructions.

2 Put the onion and olive oil in a wok or deep frying pan (skillet) and cook over a low heat for 10 minutes. Add the garlic, ginger, chilli and spices and cook gently for a further 10 minutes.

3 Meanwhile, skin the tomatoes. Cut a cross in the top of each tomato and put in a large heatproof bowl. Pour over enough boiling water to cover and leave for 10 seconds. Remove the tomatoes from the water using a slotted spoon, and peel off the skin when they are cool enough to handle. Discard the seeds and roughly chop the tomato flesh.

4 Add the chopped tomatoes and water to the onion mixture. Raise the heat to medium, bring up to a simmer and cook for 10 minutes. Allow to cool slightly then transfer to a liquidizer and blitz until smooth.

5 Put the cauliflower and sauce in a saucepan over a medium heat. Bring up to a simmer and cook for 10 minutes. Add the beans and cook for a further 3–4 minutes, until the beans are tender. Stir in the spinach and cook for 1 minute, until just wilted. Season with the grated nutmeg.

6 Drain any excess water from the rice. Serve the curry on a bed of rice, with the coriander (cilantro) sprinkled over.

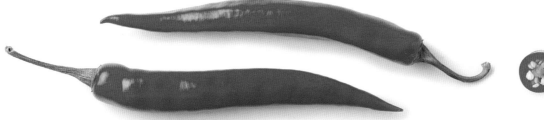

ENERGY DESSERTS

Creamy rice pudding

SERVES 1 (LARGE PORTION)
PREPARATION TIME 15 MINUTES (PLUS 40 MINUTES FOR
THE BROWN RICE)
COOKING TIME 30 MINUTES

175 ml/6oz/¾ cup rice milk
60 ml /2oz/¼ cup fresh apple juice
110g/4oz/½ cup cooked brown rice
1 tbsp raisins, chopped
1 tbsp sunflower seeds, crushed
½ tsp ground cinnamon
½ tsp organic vanilla powder, to taste

1 Combine all the ingredients, except the vanilla, in a saucepan.

2 Heat and simmer gently for 20–30 minutes, stirring often to prevent sticking. Add more rice milk if needed.

3 When the sauce is thick and creamy, stir in the vanilla. Serve warm or chilled.

Blueberries with lashings of banana sauce

SERVES 1
PREPARATION TIME 5 MINUTES

110g/4oz/½ cup fresh blueberries, washed
118 ml/4 fl oz/½ cup live, full-fat natural yogurt
½–1 tsp lemon juice
1 medium banana
½ tsp organic vanilla powder

1 In a food processor, or blender, combine all the ingredients except the blueberries. Blend until very smooth.

2 Place the blueberries in a bowl. Pour the banana cream over the blueberries and serve.

Silken fruit delight

SERVES 1
PREPARATION TIME 8 MINUTES

150g/5oz/⅔ cup light silken tofu, drained
50g/2oz/¼ cup cubed, pitted, peeled mango
50g/2oz /¼ cup strawberries, blueberries or raspberries
118 ml/4 fl oz /½ cup fresh orange juice

1 Place all the ingredients in a blender or food processor.

2 Blend until smooth, adding enough orange juice to make the desired consistency. Pour into a bowl and serve.

Macro fruit purée

SERVES 1
PREPARATION TIME 5 MINUTES
COOKING TIME 30 MINUTES

60g/2oz/¼ cup mixed, rolled organic millet and rolled organic quinoa
1 tsp unhulled tahini
230ml /8 fl oz/1 cup rice or soya (soy) milk
I tbsp seeded raisins, chopped
1 ripe pear, de-seeded and unpeeled
1 very ripe apricot
1 medium ripe banana
2 almonds, cracked

1 Place the millet and quinoa mix in a small pot. Add the raisins, tahini and milk. Cook on a medium heat, stirring regularly until creamy and well cooked.

2 Place the warm grain mixture in a bowl. Allow to cool.

3 Place the pear, banana and apricot in a blender and mix into a fine purée. Place the puréed fruit on top of the cooled grain. Garnish with the cracked almonds.

THE PURE-FOODS TOTAL CLEANSE PLAN

You've done the individual plans, and now you want to combine them in the ultimate whole-body clean out. You can do it! A totally new you begins here.

Step 1: preparation

I want to help you to make the full cleanse as easy as possible and planning is the key to success. First, clean your house from top to bottom so that all you have to do during the total cleanse is quick surface cleaning just to keep it tidy and dust-free. Enlist the help of anyone you live with to respect your communal space – you are cleaning out not only your body, but your mind and emotions too and having a fresh space to live in is fundamental.

Get your diary out and block off your total-cleanse weeks so that you do not book up too many commitments. Explain to as many of your friends and family as possible what you are doing and why you might be out of circulation for a few weeks. The plans will work best if you transition smoothly from one to the next, so read through them several times to familiarize yourself with their content and aims, and so that the basics are in your head. Keep this book somewhere handy and flag the relevant pages so that you can refer to things quickly and easily whenever you need to.

Step 2: the menu plan

You will begin the total cleanse with the month-long plan for your area of greatest need (see questionnaire, p.39), so look at this menu plan and note down in your diary, or on a wall chart, which recipes you will need each day for the first four weeks. Next you'll do the week-long plan for the area that scored second-highest. Note down the recipes you'll need each day for that week. Finally, you will do the weekend plan for the area with the lowest score, so note down these recipes for the final two days of your total cleanse. Immediately before you begin the cleanse, do a big shop to buy all the non-perishables, as well as everything you need for the first week (fresh foods are a must, so don't buy any fruits or vegetables more than a few days before you'll use them). Consider buying the supplements for detox and digestion (see pp.51 and 89) to help support the cleanse. Finally, all the rules on desserts and snacking apply to the individual plans as you do them – read up on each one and follow them accordingly.

Step 3: action

Breathing, relaxing and stretching (BRS) are crucial in the pure-foods total cleanse plan. If you have space, add the guidance given in each of the individual programs into your diary or wall chart, so that you know what BRS exercises to aim for every day. Plan to do around 20 minutes of BRS each morning and each evening (making 40 minutes each day in total). This will help you to stay focused on your cleanse as well as benefiting your body in its own ways (toning the digestive tract, enhancing the elimination systems and so on).

BRS will also add a mental and emotional aspect to your cleanse. This is especially important for the total cleanse: because the cleanse is drawn out over a longer period of time, it is likely that it will bring up, or highlight, emotional issues that you may have buried within you. BRS helps you to process and let go of accumulated emotional and mental baggage, setting you free to move on with your life and live it more fully. Try the exercise on the right if you find that your deep emotions surface during the plan. Don't try to suppress any emotions that come up – remember that negative or particularly strong emotions can be as toxic and as damaging to health as unhealthy, unnatural chemicals in your food. Welcome their surfacing and use the visualization to let them go for ever.

Exercise is an integral part of any program. Have a thorough read about exercise on pages 214–16 and plan to do a minimum of three hours a week. This could involve anything from a brisk walk in the park to an intense work-out in the gym. Aim to raise your heart rate a little, but always exercise according to your capabilities and levels of fitness.

EMOTIONAL CLEANSING VISUALIZATION

1 Ensure that you will not be disturbed – turn off your cell phone, put on the answer machine and ask friends and family to leave you alone until you emerge again. Loosen any tight clothing and lie down comfortably on a bed or on the floor. Close your eyes.

2 Imagine that you are standing at the top of a flight of ten wide stairs leading down into a beautiful sunlit glade in a forest. Walk slowly down the steps With each step feel yourself relaxing more deeply, letting go and surrendering to relaxation.

3 When you reach the bottom of the steps you see a bright white path leading toward a door. The door is surrounded by intense white light.

4 Open the door. In front of you, you see a room filled with smaller doors. Imagine light streaming through the door behind you. It beats warmly on your back, making you feel safe and supported. The light shining from this door brightly illuminates all the smaller doors in the room.

5 Each of the smaller doors leads to another room containing an incident in your life that has hurt, angered or confused you. One by one, slowly and gently, open each door and examine the incident and emotion that lies behind it. Don't linger on the emotion. Notice it and imagine the bright light flooding into the room, cleansing and healing the emotion, allowing you to forgive, forget and let go.

6 Close each door after cleansing its room with light. Feel the release of letting go of your negativity. When you have visited each room, slowly turn back toward the main entrance and walk toward the stairs. Feel your breath as you climb each step; feel the relaxation in your body. Open your eyes.

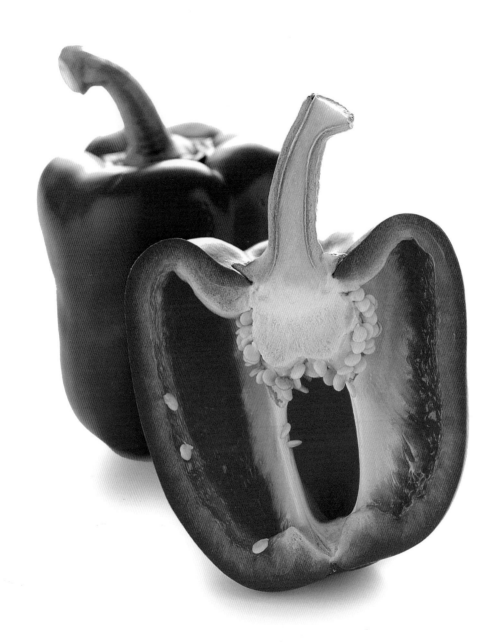

the ailment plans

Eating pure foods can help to prevent and heal a whole array of illnesses and other health complaints – from problems with your immune system, through to acne and nagging seasonal problems such as hay fever. In this chapter we take a detailed look at 14 common health conditions and suggest ways that healthy eating can help to alleviate suffering, reduce symptoms and even put us on the path to recovery. As a bonus, each ailment has a great recipe to help you make the most of your newfound knowledge about the effects of pure foods on your health.

PURE FOODS, PURE YOU – INTRODUCING THE AILMENT PLANS

Food can make you sick – we all know that too much saturated fat and refined sugar will take its toll on our heart and lungs. The great news is that food also has an amazing power to heal.

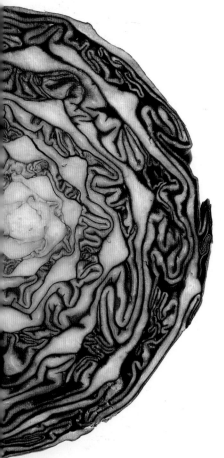

Reversing the trend

Health professionals are now certain that diabetes, cancer, arthritis, obesity and fertility problems are all on the increase as a result of poor diet. However, I want to help you by showing you how to turn all that on its head and to use pure foods to make you well if you are already ill, and to prevent illness in the first place if you aren't. We all know that vegetables are good for us, but some are better than others – some pack a mighty phytochemical (healthy, natural plant chemical) health punch! According to some recent research, a diet rich in green leafy vegetables can almost halve the risk of colon cancer. Let us take a journey through some of our veggie health allies.

Healing foods

BROCCOLI This member of the cruciferous family of vegetables is rich in antioxidants and is known to protect against colon cancer. It is also rich in indoles, a phytochemical that seems to modify the metabolism of estrogen in a woman's body, decreasing the risk of breast cancer.

TOMATOES One of the main ingredients in tomatoes is a phytochemical called lycopene, which fights cancer-causing free radicals (see p.36). This phytochemical is particularly effective in helping to prevent male prostatic cancers. Recent research has also shown that men who eat high levels of lycopene are about half as likely to have a heart attack compared with their tomato-deficient counterparts.

SPINACH Two powerful plant antioxidants in the humble spinach, lutein and zeaxanthin, seem to protect against age-related eye diseases, including cataracts and macular degeneration (a disease affecting part of the retina).

CABBAGE The humble cabbage contains plant chemicals known as indoles and sulforaphane, which are known to protect against stomach and bowel cancer. One recent US study showed that people who ate cabbage twice a week reduced their chances of contracting bowel cancer by two thirds. Its high levels of vitamin K make it excellent for preventing or easing stomach ulcers.

RED (BELL) PEPPERS Red peppers contain immune-boosting vitamin C and beta carotene. In addition all colours of pepper contain a substance called capsaicin, which is know to help keep the heart and circulation in peak condition.

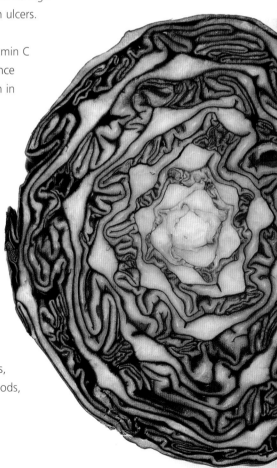

GARLIC This healthy favourite has abundant sulphur compounds that can help lower cholesterol and reduce blood clotting (easing circulation). Garlic also gently stimulates the immune system, helping us to keep well.

SHIITAKE MUSHROOMS These tasty little mushrooms contain the phytochemical lentinan, which is used as an anti-cancer drug in Japan. The benefit is thought to come from the lentinan's ability to stimulate the action of infection-fighting white blood cells in the body.

This is just a small selection of the hundreds of edible plants that nature has provided to keep us healthy. Most are common vegetables, yet they present an impressive list of health-giving properties. Pure foods, pure you!

ABDOMINAL BLOATING

Say no to sugar and allergenic foods and stock up on the friendly bacteria.

What is bloating?

There is a lot of confusion surrounding the term abdominal bloating. It does not mean water retention or fat on the belly. Bloating indicates a digestive problem and the symptoms are a distended, lower abdomen, griping pains, and flatulence. It often occurs after eating, especially certain foods, and might get progressively worse during the day.

Pure-food solutions

EAT SLOWLY Wolfing food down without giving your stomach time to realize it's coming, and failing to chew food to mix it with the digestive enzymes in your saliva, can all contribute to bloating. Remember my advice in the Digestion Tune-up? Savour your food – look at it, smell it, taste it properly, and chew it slowly.

DRINK BEFORE OR AFTER MEALS I also advised in the Digestion chapter that you didn't drink with your meals. This dilutes the digestive juices, meaning that food sits longer than it should in the stomach and intestines and begins to ferment. As the food ferments it causes wind, which in turn causes bloating. Drink before or a while after meals, but not with them. It is interesting to note that pure foods, such as fresh vegetables, contain more natural fluids and less salt than processed foods. Eating pure foods can mean that you will be a lot less thirsty during and immediately after your meals.

COMBINE FOODS Most of us can cope with a plate full of different foods. Some of us, especially those of us with stomachs weakened by a diet of poor-quality foods, can't and need to simplify our meal combinations. The stomach deals with proteins and carbohydrates very differently. It produces acid to help break down proteins and alkali to break down carbohydrates. When it has to produce both at once, because you are eating both proteins and carbohydrates in the same meal, the acid and alkali neutralize each other, delaying digestion and leaving food to ferment in the intestines. To combat this when you eat carbs, avoid protein – and vice versa (see p.90–91).

REDUCE THE ALLERGENS The body and immune system treat allergenic foods in the same way as they would a virus or bacteria. The mucous membranes lining the digestive tract go on red alert, initiating an immune reaction and producing mucus to protect you from attack. This mucus, and other protective reactions, hinder the digestive process, slowing down digestion and creating fermentation and bloating. Try to have fewer of the common allergenic foods, including wheat products, white flour, sugar, cow's dairy and alcohol. This is by no means a complete list – for example, I have a client who is allergic to kiwi fruit. Eating a wide range of pure foods tends to reduce any obvious allergenic reactions to food, easing digestion and reducing bloating. Constant focus on one particular food type will increase your chances of developing a reaction to that particular food (see p.84). If your nemesis is cow's milk, it might be an idea to rotate different dairy types in your diet. Consider trying goat's and sheep's dairy alongside cow's.

REDUCE SUGAR We have talked about fermentation in the digestive tract leading to bloating. Sugar is a fundamental part of the fermentation process, especially when it is combined with white-flour and yeast products, as in many cakes and white breads. Think how sugar and yeast work together in the fermentation process of beer and Champagne. The natural by-product of too much sugar in our diet is wind and bloating. The solution? Easy – reduce the amount of sugar you eat.

REDUCE CONSTIPATION Anything that prolongs the time it takes for food to move through the bowels is likely to lead to gas. Reduce constipation by eating fibre-rich pure foods, such as wholemeal rye pasta and fresh vegetables, drinking more water, massaging your lower abdomen (see p.93) and having the occasional colonic irrigation if the problem is bad. Laxatives are not a solution. The Digestion tune-up plan in Chapter 3 will work wonders.

BEAT STRESS As we learned in Chapter 3, stress diverts blood away from the digestive process, slowing down digestion, and once again leaving food to ferment in the intestine. Pure foods such as wholegrain millet and fresh eggs are rich in the B-vitamins, which help to calm the nervous system and correct the damage caused by the stress of modern life.

INCREASE GOOD BACTERIA The hot topic in the world of bowels is the "good bacteria" – beneficial flora or probiotics (see pp.82–4). When one or more of these bacteria grow out of control they become "bad bacteria" and start to impact negatively on digestion. A diet rich in simple sugars and low in fibre is the perfect breeding ground for some of the less beneficial bowel flora. Good bacteria are found in abundance in healthy, fermented pure foods, such as natural live yogurt and kefir. Note that antibiotics can reduce the numbers of good bacteria in the bowel, so optimizing your immune system can also have an impact on the likelihood of developing abdominal bloating.

Supplements to beat abdominal bloating

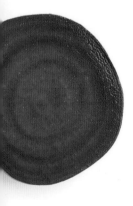

- Lactobacillus acidophilus and bifidus are the main "friendly" bacteria in our bowels. These probiotics stabilize digestion and help in the metabolism of the B-vitamins, which ease the nervous system and regulate blood sugars.
- A great first-aid technique for bloating is to use digestive enzyme capsules. These contain the enzymes necessary for the breakdown and digestion of the proteins, fats, plant fibre, and carbohydrates in our diets. Digestive enzymes can reduce bloating significantly, but it does pay to remember that they are not fixing the underlying problem of a weak digestive tract.
- Two medicinal herbs are renowned for their beneficial effects on digestion and, specifically, bloating. Peppermint stimulates the release of digestive enzymes, speeding up the process of food through the digestive system and helping to reduce fermentation and wind. Fennel is a wonderful digestive and will settle the stomach, reduce wind and soothe away indigestion. Take either of these herbs as a delicious herbal tea after a meal.

Tray-baked trout with beetroot (beet) relish

SERVES 2
PREPARATION TIME 10 MINUTES
COOKING TIME 35–40 MINUTES

1 medium bulb fennel (300g/11oz), sliced into
8 from top to root

4 tsp extra virgin olive oil

½ tsp fresh thyme leaves

2 x 300g/11oz whole organic trout, gutted and cleaned

1 medium lemon, cut into 8 wedges

1 medium cooked beetroot (beet) (80g/3oz),
peeled and diced

4 tbsp live goat's yogurt

1   Heat the oven to 180°C/fan160°C/350°F/gas 4.

2   Put the fennel, 3 tsp olive oil and the thyme in a large bowl and turn the fennel in the oil until well coated. Lay the fennel slices on a large baking sheet and cook in the top part of the oven for 15 minutes.

3   Insert two lemon wedges into the cavity of each trout. Turn the fennel slices over and lay the trout on top, then drizzle over the remaining olive oil. Return to the oven and bake for 20–25 minutes, until the fish is cooked through.

4   Meanwhile, mix the beetroot (beet) and yogurt together in a small bowl. Transfer the trout and fennel to two plates and serve with the beetroot relish and remaining lemon wedges.

NOTES: If you use trout fillets, bake the fennel for 15 minutes, turn and bake for a further 15 minutes. Lay the trout fillets on top, brush with olive oil and cook for 7–8 minutes, until the fish is cooked through.

You can use boiled cooked beetroot (beet) (not pickled) from the supermarket. To roast beetroot, follow the recipe for Roast salmon and beetroot (beet) salad on page 74.

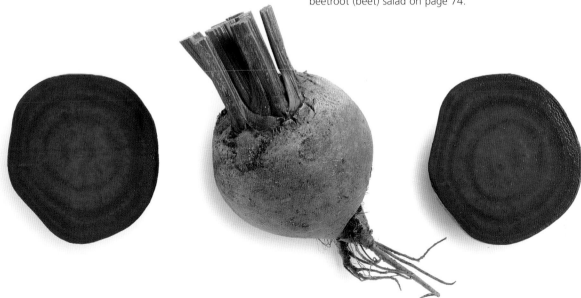

ACNE

Eat pure foods rich in zinc, fibre, essential fatty acids and vitamin A.

What is acne?

The medical definition of acne is that it is an "inflammatory sebaceous skin disease with pustules, papules and cysts". The sebaceous glands, found in each hair follicle, produce oil that lubricates the skin. If the oil becomes trapped in the gland, bacteria begin to breed, causing a spot. Blackheads occur when the oil, or sebum, in the gland mixes with coloured skin pigments and plugs the pore. Whiteheads are a sign that the oil has spread under the skin, building up and causing inflammation and pain. The whitehead can become infected with bacteria, causing further discomfort and angst.

Pure-food solutions

REDUCE TOXINS Naturopaths place the blame for acne primarily at the door of poor diet and the increase in toxins this represents. Refined sugars, saturated animal fats, hydrogenated oil, rancid oils, pesticides, preservatives and colourings are all forms of dietary toxin. Unless we eliminate these toxins, via the liver, the kidneys, the lungs, the bowels and the skin, they accumulate in our blood. The skin then bears the brunt of the toxic overload. The body forces toxins out onto the skin surface where they can no longer cause any internal damage. Cleaning up your diet is crucial to minimize your susceptibility to acne. A diet rich in whole grains, fruits and vegetables ensures a good supply of the top skin nutrients, including the mineral zinc and vitamin A, which have antibacterial properties, and essential fatty acids (EFAs). Zinc is found in abundance in raw nuts, mushrooms and pumpkin seeds; vitamin A in corn and salmon. EFAs are found in oily fish, such as tuna and salmon, and cold-pressed vegetable oils. Make sure you get plenty of fibre, to keep your digestive system working optimally, eliminating toxins through your bowels. Try not to use any salt in your diet, especially iodized salt. Iodine has been shown to worsen acne.

BALANCE THE HORMONES A hormone imbalance or a sudden surge of hormones (for example, at puberty, or post-ovulation in a woman) can also cause acne. Modern, processed foods contain chemicals that can interfere with the body's own natural hormonal balance. Eating organic meat, poultry and fish reduces your exposure to these troublesome synthetic substances.

Warm wild rice salad with griddled tuna

SERVES 2
PREPARATION TIME 15 MINUTES (PLUS OVERNIGHT SOAKING)
COOKING TIME 50 MINUTES

2 tbsp aduki beans
30g/1oz/¼ cup wild rice
55g/2oz/⅓ cup brown rice
1 bay leaf
6 salad onions, trimmed and finely sliced

3 tbsp pumpkin seeds, lightly toasted
Small bunch coriander (cilantro), chopped
1 tsp lime juice
2 tsp sesame oil
2 tsp extra virgin olive oil
2 x 150g/5oz line-caught yellow fin tuna steaks, 5cm/2in thick
2 lime quarters, to serve

1 Soak the beans overnight. Rinse and put them into a saucepan with cold water to cover the beans by 1cm/½in. Bring to the boil and cook for 10 minutes. Drain, rinse, and return to the pan with the wild and brown rice and bay.

2 Add enough water to cover the rice and beans by 5cm/2in. Over a medium heat, simmer and cook for 45 minutes, adding extra water if it gets too dry. Drain and remove the bay leaf.

3 Tip the rice salad into a medium bowl and stir in the onions, pumpkin seeds, coriander (cilantro), lime juice and sesame and olive oils.

4 Preheat a griddle pan. Griddle the tuna for 1 minute (rare) or 2 minutes (medium-rare) on each side. Divide the salad between two plates and top with the tuna. Serve with the lime.

ASTHMA

Eat plenty of magnesium-rich pure foods and reduce your intake of cow's dairy.

What is asthma?

Asthma is caused by spasms in the bronchial passages, which restrict the flow of air in and out of the lungs. The mucous membranes that line the bronchi become inflamed, overproducing mucus and restricting air-flow still further. Dust, pollution, food additives and stress are among the many asthma triggers.

Pure-food solutions

REDUCE COW'S DAIRY The allergenic proteins in milk irritate the lining of the lungs and bronchioles, forcing the body to release histamine, which causes inflammation and increased mucus. Try goat's or sheep's milk instead.

INCREASE VITAMINS C AND A Vitamin C is a natural antihistamine, so eat plenty of fruits and vegetables. Vitamin A (in blueberries, corn, yellow fruits, and tomatoes) will repair lung tissue and boost immunity.

INCREASE EFAS Essential fatty acids (see p.202) help the body to produce anti-inflammatories called prostaglandins. This reduces inflammation in the bronchi, helping to prevent the onset of an attack.

INCREASE MAGNESIUM Magnesium (whole grains, beans, dark green vegetables, fish and kiwi) helps to reduce spasms in the bronchial passages.

Grilled (broiled) chicken with nutty millet pilaf

SERVES 2
PREPARATION TIME 20 MINUTES
COOKING TIME 35 MINUTES

55g/2oz/⅓ cup millet
200ml/7 fl oz/⅞ cup vegetable stock
¼ tsp ground allspice
2 shallots (scallions) (30g/1oz), peeled and thinly sliced
2 tbsp extra virgin olive oil

1 tbsp unsalted cashew nuts, chopped and lightly toasted
2 x 110g/4oz skinless, boneless organic chicken breasts
2 heads pak choi (200g /7oz), halved
Very small bunch flat leaf parsley, chopped
2 lemon quarters, to serve

1 Put the millet in a small bowl and cover with boiling water. Leave to soak for 10 minutes.

2 Drain the millet and put in a medium saucepan with the stock and allspice. Place over a medium heat and bring up to a simmer. Cook for 20 minutes, adding a little extra stock if the millet gets too dry.

3 Meanwhile, put the shallots (scallions) and 1 tbsp olive oil in a frying pan (skillet) over a low heat. Cook gently for 15–20 minutes until the shallots are soft and golden. Stir occasionally to prevent them from burning. Stir the shallots (scallions) and cashew nuts into the millet and keep warm.

4 Preheat the grill (broiler) to high. Put the chicken breasts between two large pieces of greaseproof paper and use a rolling pin to flatten the breasts into escalopes about 1cm/½in thick. Brush with the remaining olive oil and grill (broil) the chicken breasts for 3–4 minutes on each side, until cooked through.

5 Steam the pak choi for 3–4 minutes, until tender. Stir the parsley into the millet pilaff and divide between two plates. Add the chicken and pak choi and serve with lemon quarters.

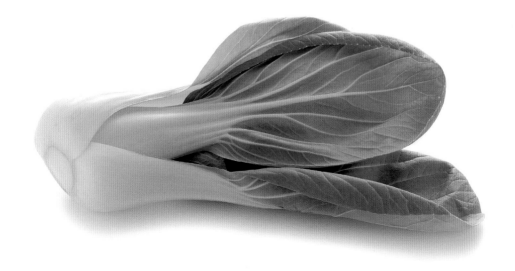

ECZEMA

Eat foods rich in essential fatty acids, alkalize the blood with fresh fruits and vegetables, and eat less red meat.

What is eczema?

Eczema is an inflammation of the skin with redness, scales and thickening, and most often fluid-filled blisters that can ooze and crack. The most common causes seem to be allergies (external reactions to perfumes, cosmetics, jewelry and in some cases internal reactions to food) and stress. It can be hereditary.

Pure-food solutions

INCREASE EFAS Your body needs essential fatty acids (see p.202) to build new cells and repair those that are damaged, especially in your skin. It also needs them to produce prostaglandins, which reduce inflammation and so will help to soothe the discomfort of eczema. The body is unable to manufacture EFAs, so they must come from food. There are two basic types: omega-3 and, most important for treating eczema, omega-6. Try taking a mix of omega-3 and omega-6 in capsule or liquid form as a daily supplement.

INCREASE ALKALIZING FOODS All of the biochemical reactions in the body require a stable pH or acid–alkaline balance in the body to function normally. Sugar, caffeine, meat, alcohol, refined white flour and stress tend to push us toward an acidic state, in which eczema will flourish. Alkalizing the body reduces inflammation and can have a marked impact on the redness and heat associated with eczema. See page 203 for a list of the top alkalizing foods and increase these in your diet.

AVOID ALLERGENS Food allergies compromise immune function, creating inflammation and chemical reactions in the body that can lead to or worsen eczema. Cow's dairy and wheat are major culprits – avoid them.

EASE LIVER FUNCTION The liver eliminates toxins. If it is overworked, it produces excess heat, which is released onto the skin, creating inflammation, leading to eczema. Try the detox plans (Chapter 2) to ease the liver's load.

Sesame-crusted salmon with stir-fried kale

SERVES 2
PREPARATION TIME 10 MINUTES
COOKING TIME 10 MINUTES

2 tsp extra virgin olive oil

2 x 170g/6oz organic salmon fillets, skin on

2 tbsp sesame seeds, lightly toasted

1 clove garlic, peeled and crushed

½ tsp fresh ginger, grated

6 handfuls kale leaves (6oz/170g), torn into bite-sized pieces

¼ red chilli, seeds removed and finely chopped

2 tbsp water

2 tsp wheat-free tamari

2 lime quarters, to serve

1 Preheat the oven to 200°C/fan 180°C/400°F/ gas 6.

2 Brush 1 tsp of the olive oil on to the flesh side of the salmon fillets. Sprinkle the sesame seeds on a plate, then press the oiled side of the salmon into the seeds. Put the salmon on a lightly oiled baking sheet, sesame-coated-side up, and roast in the top of the oven for 7–8 minutes, until the fish is cooked.

3 Meanwhile, pour the remaining olive oil into a wok and place over a medium heat. Add the garlic and ginger and cook for 30 seconds, then add the kale, chilli and water and stir-fry for 5–6 minutes. Stir in the tamari and cook for a further minute, then remove from the heat.

4 Divide the stir-fry between two plates and top with the salmon. Serve with lime quarters.

HAY FEVER (ALLERGIC RHINITIS)

Eat foods rich in immune-boosting vitamins C and E, and avoid cow's dairy.

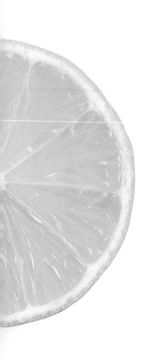

What is hay fever?

An overactive immune system may identify pollen or other airborne particles as pathogens. These irritate the mucous membranes lining the nose and sinuses so that they produce watery mucus to flush away the offending particles. The body also releases histamines, which cause inflammation in the sinuses.

Pure-food solutions

AVOID ALLERGENIC FOODS Try to avoid typical allergens, which will exacerbate the immune response, especially the production of mucus. Wheat and cow's dairy are the main culprits.

EAT MORE RAW FRUIT AND VEG Eat lots of organic fruit and vegetables high in antioxidants, such as vitamins A, C and E and the mineral zinc, to stabilize the immune system. The richest antioxidant foods are the berry family.

AVOID INFLAMMATORY FOODS Red meat and eggs contain a compound called arachidonic acid (AA), too much of which exacerbates inflammation. Deadly nightshades (see p.184) can also make inflammation worse.

EAT LOCAL HONEY Local honey contains pollen local to your area. It can acclimatize your immune system to the pollen, reducing the immune response.

Rice paper rolls with ginger citrus dipping sauce

MAKES 24
PREPARATION TIME 45 MINUTES
COOKING TIME 4 MINUTES

110g/4oz skinless organic chicken breast, cut into thin strips

1 tbsp extra virgin olive oil

1 fat clove garlic, peeled and crushed

½ green apple, peeled, cored and cut into matchsticks

4 salad onions, trimmed and cut into thin strips lengthways

½ red (bell) pepper, cut into matchsticks

3 large Chinese leaf leaves, stems discarded and leaves finely shredded

¼ medium cucumber (85g/3oz), cut into matchsticks

Small bunch coriander (cilantro), chopped

20 mint leaves, shredded

24 rice paper roll wrappers

3 tbsp fresh orange juice

4 tsp lime or lemon juice

1 tsp fresh ginger, grated

¼ red chilli, finely chopped (optional)

1 Put the chicken, olive oil and garlic into a wok over a high heat and stir-fry for 3–4 minutes, until cooked through. Spread out on a plate and leave to cool for 10 minutes.

2 Put the apple, onions, pepper, Chinese leaf, cucumber, coriander (cilantro) and mint into a large bowl. Add the cooled chicken, plus any juices on the plate, and toss together thoroughly.

3 Pour about 1.5cm/¾in cold water in a shallow dish. Dip a rice paper wrapper in the water and leave for 2 minutes to soften. Remove and spread out on a dry tea towel. Put a heaped teaspoon of the filling on the edge of the wrapper closest to you and fold the side edges inward to enclose the filling, then roll up.

4 Dampen the opposite edge of the rice paper wrapper slightly and press down to seal the roll, then put on a plate, seam side down, and cover with damp kitchen paper. Repeat with the remaining rice paper wrappers and filling.

5 To make the dipping sauce, mix the orange juice, lime juice, ginger and chilli in a small bowl. Uncover the finished rolls and serve with the dipping sauce.

NOTE: You can wrap the filling in little gem lettuce leaves rather than rice paper if you want to avoid carbohydrates. Vegetarians can replace the chicken with 3 tbsp chopped and lightly toasted unsalted cashew nuts or peanuts.

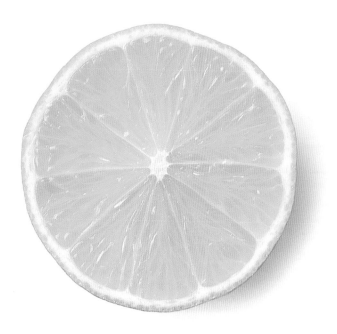

HEADACHES

Eat foods rich in the amino acid L-tryptophan and in magnesium.

What are headaches?

There are many different types of headache: exertion, caffeine, fever, sinus, cluster and migraine among them. The most common, the tension headache, is generally caused by muscle tension altering blood-flow to the brain. Other causes can be teeth-grinding, sinus congestion, infection, dehydration, and poor alignment of the spine. In addition, naturopaths see food allergies, high blood pressure, bowel problems and low blood sugars as common triggers.

Pure-food solutions

REDUCE FOOD ALLERGENS Frequent, unexplained headaches might be a sign of food sensitivity. Turn to a pure foods diet, eating only freshly prepared meals and staying away from the unnatural chemicals in processed, packaged foods. Keeping a food diary (see p.91) may help to identify possible triggers.

EAT LESS SALT Raised blood pressure (BP) is a common cause of headaches, especially the early-morning variety. One of the main food culprits of high BP is salt. Move to a low- or no-salt diet.

EAT MORE FIBRE A regular bowel motion ensures that the toxins in your stool are released from the body. If you are constipated, waste sits in the lower intestines and creates toxic headaches. Eat regular daily portions of fibre-rich foods, such as brown rice, prunes, beans, lentils and fresh raw vegetables.

EAT LOW-GI FOODS Sugar in your blood gives you energy. Any sharp drop in blood sugars can trigger a headache. Low-GI foods (see pp.120–121) offer a steady release of sugar into the blood, and therefore fewer headaches.

EAT MORE MAGNESIUM The mineral magnesium helps to maintain the correct function of nerves and muscles. A deficiency can contribute to tension headaches. Apples, apricots and brown rice are all rich in magnesium.

BOOST L-TRYPTOPHAN This essential amino acid helps transfer nerve impulses from one cell to another. It assists with the proper functioning of the nervous system and can reduce the muscle spasms that cause headaches. Food sources include brown rice, cottage cheese and soya (soy).

Lemon-baked halibut with garlic-braised chicory

SERVES 2
PREPARATION TIME 15 MINUTES
COOKING TIME 40 MINUTES

2 heads chicory (180g/6oz), quartered
1 fat clove garlic, peeled and crushed
100ml/3 fl oz/½ cup vegetable stock

2 x 170g/6oz Pacific halibut steaks
½ medium lemon, very thinly sliced
2 tbsp chopped almonds, lightly toasted

1 Preheat the oven to 200°C/fan 180°C/400°F/gas 6.

2 Place the chicory in a single layer on the bottom of a baking dish. Whisk the garlic into the vegetable stock and pour over the chicory. Bake for 30 minutes, turning the chicory over halfway through. Add a little extra stock if the dish becomes dry.

3 Sit the halibut steaks on top of the chicory and lay the lemon slices over the top of the fish. Return to the oven and cook for a further 8–10 minutes, until the fish is just cooked.

4 Carefully transfer the halibut to two plates using a fish slice. Sprinkle the toasted almonds over the chicory before serving. Press the flesh of the lemon slices with a knife to squeeze any remaining juice into the halibut, then lift off and discard.

NOTE: If you would prefer to eat the fish with a chicory salad, bake the lemon-topped halibut steaks on a lightly oiled baking sheet for 8–10 minutes. Serve the chicory leaves with a dressing made from 2 tbsp olive oil and 2 tsp lemon juice and with the toasted almonds sprinkled over.

IMMUNITY

Beat the bugs: eat pure foods rich in vitamin C, lymph-friendly zinc and vitamin A, and the antioxidant selenium.

What is the immune system?

Your wonderful immune system is your protection against anything that poses a threat to your body. These threats are known as antigens, and an antigen may be anything from bacteria and viruses through to chemical food additives. The immune system identifies the threat, works out how to deal with it, then remembers the process – that's how we acquire immunity against viruses and bacteria, so once you've had, say, chickenpox once, you are unlikely to catch it again. The attacking end of the immune system is provided by your white blood cells. These travel the blood stream, seeking out and destroying antigens.

However, the immune system is not without its weakness and it can function properly only if it gets all the nutrients it needs for maximum effectiveness. This means packing your body full with vitamin C and with antioxidants, such as vitamin E and the minerals zinc and selenium. In addition, we should take steps to reduce the factors that depress immune function. These include foods that we might be sensitive or allergic to, which send the immune system into overdrive, attacking perfectly harmless foods (commonly wheat-based and dairy products) as antigens. Stress, poor lymphatic function, and an overload of pollution, free radicals (see p.36) and chemical toxins also place unnecessary strain on your immune system, causing it to malfunction and leaving you prone to colds, flu and a host of other ailments, minor and major.

Pure-food solutions

BOOST THE VITAMIN C Quite simply, your immune system loves vitamin C. It helps to fight off viruses, bacteria and free radicals; it also helps to detoxify the body, beat back allergens and boost the lymphatic system, which manufactures and stores the all-important white blood cells. In addition, foods rich in vitamin C help the body to cope with the negative effects of stress, including its weakening effects on white blood cells. Aim for two daily portions of some of the following vitamin C-rich pure foods: green leafy vegetables, green and red (bell) peppers, broccoli, cauliflower, Brussels sprouts, kiwi, berries, green peas, and tomatoes.

EAT MORE VITAMIN A AND ZINC Vitamin A and zinc are crucial for the proper manufacture of T-cells – the killer white blood cells that launch a direct attack on pathogens. Vitamin A (in the form of beta-carotene) is found in red and orange foods, such as cantaloupe melons, mangoes, red (bell) peppers, carrots and butternut squash. Spinach, eggs and wholemeal corn porridge are also good sources. Get your boost of zinc in the form of ground-up pumpkin seeds sprinkled over your salads. Or eat more lentils, chickpeas (garbanzos) or brown rice.

EAT MORE SELENIUM Selenium is a powerful mineral antioxidant, protecting the body against the cancer-causing free radicals. In addition it supports the immune system, helping it to perform optimally in its fight against disease. It is great for detoxifying the body and also helping to reduce inflammation (often the first sign that the immune system is activating). Selenium-rich foods include mushrooms, sunflower seeds and Brazil nuts.

EAT MORE GARLIC Garlic is the ultimate immune food. It has a long history as an immune-booster, and countless scientific studies have shown that it improves the activity of the immune system. It is antiviral and antifungal, so makes the perfect addition to any immune-boosting diet. If you are worried about the smell of garlic on your breath, or don't particularly like the flavour, crush the garlic and then heat it a little, or leave it to stand for a few hours, before you use it. When you heat or leave the garlic, the allicin, which gives the clove its pungent smell and taste, breaks down, taking away the strong smell and taste. Allicin is not the immune-boosting component of garlic, so you get the benefit without the embarrassment.

EAT OR DRINK MORE GINGER Ginger is a fabulous, warming herb that improves circulation, thus sending the white blood cells to where they are most needed. It ensures a robust response to a viral or bacterial attack. Add it to your foods, or have a regular cup of ginger tea.

EAT YOGURT EVERY DAY A daily serving of live-culture yogurt (goat's, sheep's or cow's) can help to restore the friendly bacteria (probiotics; see p.82) in your gut. The good bacteria oust any damaging bacteria, improving digestion and the absorption of other immune-boosting nutrients.

Pumpkin boulangère with roast chicken and little gem salad

SERVES 2
PREPARATION TIME 25 MINUTES
COOKING TIME 45 MINUTES

1 tbsp plus 1 tsp extra virgin olive oil
½ small pumpkin (350g/12oz of pumpkin), peeled, thinly sliced
1 small onion, peeled and thinly sliced
½ tsp fresh thyme, chopped
½ tsp fresh oregano, chopped

I clove garlic, peeled and crushed
100ml/4 fl oz/½ cup vegetable stock or water
30g/1oz/¼ cup hard goat's cheese, grated
2 x 250g/9oz organic chicken breast quarters, skin on
1 little gem lettuce, shredded
6 radishes, sliced
1 tsp cider vinegar

1 Preheat the oven to 200°C/fan 180°C/400°F/ gas 6. Oil an 850ml/1½-pint ovenproof dish with 1 tsp olive oil. Layer one third of the pumpkin slices in the base and top with half the onion. Sprinkle over half the herbs, then repeat with another layer of pumpkin, onion and herbs. Finish with pumpkin.

2 Whisk the crushed garlic into the stock and pour into the dish. Sprinkle over the cheese and bake in the top part of the oven for 10 minutes.

3 Add the chicken to the pumpkin dish in the oven and cook for 35–40 minutes, until the chicken is cooked through and the vegetables are soft.

4 Meanwhile, put the lettuce and radish in a bowl. Whisk the remaining 1 tbsp olive oil and the cider vinegar together in a bowl, then pour over the salad and toss well. Serve the chicken and pumpkin together with the salad on the side.

Dover sole with shiitake sauce and gingered greens

SERVES 2

PREPARATION TIME 40 MINUTES (INCLUDING SOAKING)
COOKING TIME 25 MINUTES

6 dried shiitake mushrooms

150ml/5 fl oz/⅔ cup boiling water

1 tbsp plus 1 tsp extra virgin olive oil

1 small shallot (scallion), peeled and finely chopped

8 fresh shiitake mushrooms, sliced

1 tsp wheat-free tamari

1 225g/8oz Dover sole fillet, skin removed

1 fat clove garlic, peeled and crushed

1 tsp fresh ginger, grated

6–8 asparagus spears, trimmed, cut to 2.5cm/1in lengths

2 tbsp water

1 head pak choi (100g/4oz)

Large handful spinach (55g/2oz)

2 lime quarters, to serve

1   Soak the dried mushrooms in boiling water for 30 minutes. Preheat the oven to 200°C/fan 180°C/400°F/gas 6.

2   Remove the mushrooms, reserving the liquid, and slice thinly. Pour 1 tsp olive oil into a frying pan (skillet) with the shallot (scallion) and soaked mushrooms. Cook over a medium heat for 5 minutes, then add the soaking liquid. Simmer for 5 minutes, reducing the liquid by two thirds. Add the fresh shiitake and simmer for a further 3–4 minutes. Stir in the tamari.

3   Lay the sole fillets in the base of an ovenproof dish and pour over the mushroom sauce. Cover with dampened greaseproof paper and bake for 8–9 minutes, until the fish is just cooked.

4   Meanwhile, pour the remaining 1 tbsp olive oil into a wok and add the garlic, ginger, asparagus and 2 tbsp water. Stir-fry over a high heat for 5 minutes, then add the pak choi and spinach and cook for 2 minutes.

5   Transfer the sole fillets to two plates and spoon over the mushroom sauce. Divide the greens between the plates and serve with the lime.

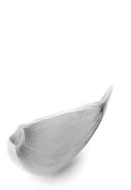
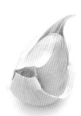
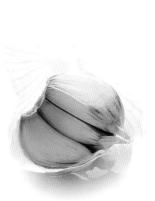
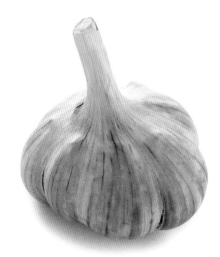

INSOMNIA

Sleep well with foods rich in magnesium, vitamin C and vitamin B5.

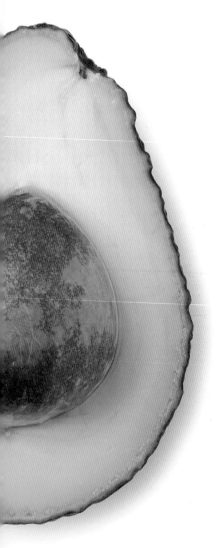

What is insomnia?

Insomnia is persistent sleeplessness. We all know the scenario of tossing and turning all through the night after a particularly stressful period at work. If this goes on for weeks and months, you may be an insomniac. Eating or working too late, drinking alcohol, taking too little exercise, adrenal exhaustion owing to stress, and yo-yoing blood-sugar levels (see p.120) can all cause insomnia.

Pure-food solutions

EAT BEFORE EIGHT When you eat too late you lie in bed digesting and not resting. This can keep you awake. Ideally you should eat at least three hours before going to bed. In addition, you can speed up digestion by food combining – separating your proteins and your carbs (see p.125).

EAT MORE STRESS-REDUCING FOODS Foods rich in vitamins C and B5 and in magnesium feed your depleted adrenals (which produce adrenaline [epinephrine]), helping to restore sleep. Broccoli, Brussels sprouts, citrus fruit, guava, kale, parsley and squash are all rich in vitamin C. Whole grains, dark green vegetables, avocadoes, fresh fish and apples are all magnesium-rich. Organic eggs, fresh fish, whole grains, nuts and all fresh fruit are rich in B5.

EAT LOW-GI FOODS High-GI (glycemic index; see p.120) foods raise the amount of sugar in your blood quickly. When the blood-sugar levels fall during the night, you wake up slightly hungry. Eating low-GI foods for dinner helps to keep your blood sugars stable, ensuring a better night's sleep.

Quinoa tart with avocado salad

SERVES 2
PREPARATION TIME 20 MINUTES
COOKING TIME 30 MINUTES (PLUS 10 MINUTES COOLING)

55g/2oz/⅓ cup quinoa, rinsed thoroughly

2 tbsp extra virgin olive oil

250g/9oz/¾ cup quark

2 large organic, free-range eggs, lightly beaten

2 fat garlic cloves, peeled and crushed

6 salad onions, trimmed and thinly sliced

Small bunch parsley, chopped

85g/3oz/¾ cup hard goat's cheese, finely grated

1 little gem lettuce or ½ cos (romaine) lettuce, shredded

1 small avocado, peeled, stoned and sliced

2 tsp lemon juice

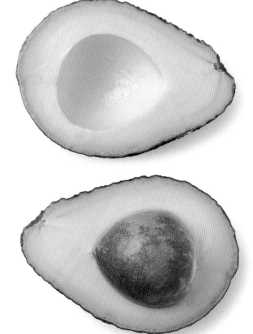

1 Cook the quinoa according to the packet instructions. Spread out on a plate and allow to cool for 10 minutes.

2 Preheat the oven to 180°C/fan 160°C/350°F/gas 4. Generously oil a 20cm/8in ovenproof pie dish or springform cake tin using half the olive oil.

3 Put the quark in a medium bowl and stir a couple of times to soften. Beat in the eggs using a wooden spoon – don't worry if they look a bit curdled at first, just keep mixing and they will combine. Then stir in the garlic, onions, parsley and cheese.

4 Spoon the mixture into the prepared dish and smooth the top. Bake in the middle of the oven for 25–30 minutes until set. Remove from the oven and allow to stand for 10 minutes before loosening the edges with a spatula and removing the tart from the dish.

5 Meanwhile, put the lettuce and avocado in a medium bowl. Whisk the remaining olive oil and the lemon juice together in a small bowl, then pour over the salad and toss well. Serve with wedges of the tart.

NOTE: If you want to brown the top of the tart, place it under a hot grill (broiler) for 2–3 minutes.

IRRITABLE BOWEL SYNDROME

Remove all allergenic foods and eat plenty of fibre-rich pure foods and natural ferments, such as yogurt and kefir.

What is irritable bowel syndrome (IBS)?

IBS is the disturbance of the rhythmic muscular contraction of the bowel, so that the stool takes longer to make its way out of the body. The blocked stool traps wind and mucus (which causes bloating) and irritates the mucous membranes lining the bowels, leading to localized inflammation. Symptoms include flatulence, nausea, and constipation and diarrhea. IBS can lead to gall-bladder disease, diabetes, arthritis and candidiasis. Causes of IBS include food allergies, low levels of probiotics, a low-fibre diet and mineral deficiency.

Pure-food solutions

ROTATE YOUR FOOD Eat a broad range of foods in rotation to reduce your exposure to potential food allergens, particularly to wheat-based foods. Rye, millet, oats, amaranth, buckwheat and quinoa are good alternatives to wheat.

EAT MORE GOOD BACTERIA We have "good" and "bad" bacteria in our intestines. The good bacteria help us to digest our food and keep the bad bacteria at bay. Regular doses of antibiotics and diets rich in simple sugars favour the growth of bad bacteria, creating indigestion and flatulence. Eating fermented foods, such as yogurt and kefir, helps to recolonize the bowels with the friendly bacteria, reducing abdominal discomfort.

EAT MORE FIBRE Fibre bulks out the stool, allowing the intestines to grip it and push it through, thus preventing constipation. Eat a plate of raw or lightly steamed vegetables and a few pieces of fruit every day. Dried prunes, nuts and seeds are all rich in fibre too.

INCREASE MAGNESIUM AND CALCIUM These minerals calm and regulate the muscles of the bowels. Magnesium-rich foods include grapefruit, green leafy vegetables, millet, avocadoes, peaches and black-eye beans. Take a regular calcium–magnesium supplement (2 parts calcium to 1 part magnesium).

Spinach and lemon falafel with mint dip

SERVES 2
PREPARATION TIME 20 MINUTES (PLUS OVERNIGHT SOAKING AND REFRIGERATION TIME)
COOKING TIME 1 HOUR 45 MINUTES (INCLUDES 1 HOUR 30 MINUTES COOKING TIME FOR CHICKPEAS [GARBANZOS])

110g/4oz/¾ cup chickpeas (garbanzos)
1 medium onion, peeled and chopped
2 tbsp extra virgin olive oil

2 fat cloves garlic, peeled and crushed
½ tsp ground cumin
½ tsp ground coriander
⅛ tsp cayenne pepper (or to taste)
2 large handfuls (110g/4oz) spinach
Juice and finely grated zest of 1 medium unwaxed lemon
6 tbsp live goat's yogurt
Small bunch mint, finely chopped

1 Soak the chickpeas (garbanzos) overnight, then cook according to the packet instructions. Drain thoroughly and allow to cool slightly.

2 Meanwhile, put the onion and 1 tbsp olive oil in a large frying pan (skillet) or wok and place over a medium heat. Cook for 5 minutes, then add the garlic and spices and continue to cook for a further 5 minutes, stirring occasionally. Add the spinach and cook for a final 5 minutes, until any liquid from the spinach has evaporated.

3 Put the chickpeas (garbanzos) and spinach mix into a food processor and add the lemon zest and 2 tsp lemon juice. Blitz to make a smooth paste. Turn the mixture into a large bowl and use your hands to form into six patties. Refrigerate for at least an hour to firm up, if possible, although you can cook the falafel straightaway if needed.

4 Put the yogurt, mint and 1 tbsp lemon juice into a small bowl and mix well.

5 Preheat the grill (broiler) to high. Brush the falafel with the remaining olive oil and grill (broil) for 3–4 minutes on each side, until golden brown. Serve the falafel with the yogurt dip on the side.

MOOD SWINGS AND DEPRESSION

Eat pure foods rich in B-vitamins, essential fatty acids and the amino acid L-tyrosine.

What are mood swings and depression?

Mood swings tend to have a cause. SAD (Seasonal Affective Disorder), brought on by the onset of winter, is a classic example; as are the mood swings brought on by fluctuating blood-sugar levels. Depression affects your nervous system, your endocrine system and your understanding of the world. There are three main types: unipolar (which generally eases with or without treatment), bipolar (alternating bursts of depression and manic activity) and low-grade but constant (feeling down, but living fairly normally). Diet, lifestyle and mental and emotional upheavals can all affect out state of mind, perhaps leading to depression, but the precise causes are not certain.

Pure-foods solutions

BOOST YOUR NUTRIENTS Thoughts are biochemical reactions facilitated by nutrients such as L-tyrosine (an amino acid found in lima beans, almonds, bananas, avocadoes and pumpkin seeds), zinc, vitamin B-complex, choline (in eggs and red and organ meat) and calcium. Also stock up on the omega-3 fish oils found in salmon and tuna; and eat plenty of raw vegetables, and fruit.

STABILIZE YOUR BLOOD SUGAR To stabilize your blood sugars eat whole grains and stay away from sugary foods. The mineral chromium (in brown rice, mushrooms, eggs and dried beans) can balance the way you metabolize sugar. Avoid caffeine, alcohol, wheat and fried foods – the "downers".

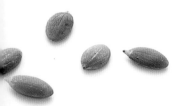

REDUCE THE ALLERGENS Some foods trigger an immune reaction because the body sees them as harmful (see p.84). According to some experts, your immune and nervous systems and your brain are closely linked – a problem with one can lead to problems in the others. So, a weak immune system may cause a tired nervous system, which may in turn leave you susceptible to depression or mood swings. Cut out the common food allergens, such as wheat and cow's dairy.

Turkey lemongrass skewers with mango rice

SERVES 2
PREPARATION TIME 15 MINUTES
*COOKING TIME 45 MINUTES (INCLUDES 30 MINUTES
MARINATING TIME FOR TURKEY)*

¼ red chilli, seeds removed and chopped

1 small clove garlic, peeled

1 tsp fresh ginger, grated

2 tsp sesame oil

2 tsp lime juice

225g/8oz skinless organic turkey breast, cut into 1cm/½in cubes

110g/4oz/⅔ cup brown rice

2 long sticks lemongrass

½ medium mango, flesh diced

2 tbsp unsalted cashew nuts, chopped and lightly toasted

2 sprigs mint, chopped

2 lime quarters, to serve

1 Put the chilli, garlic and ginger into a mortar and pound to a paste using the pestle. Transfer to a medium bowl and stir in the sesame oil and lime juice.

2 Add the turkey cubes and leave to marinate for 30 minutes. Meanwhile, cook the rice according to the packet instructions.

3 Preheat the grill (broiler) to high. Use a skewer to make a hole in the middle of each turkey cube and thread the cubes onto the lemongrass sticks. Brush on any marinade left in the bowl, then grill (broil) the skewers for 4–5 minutes on each side, until cooked through.

4 Drain the rice and stir in the mango, cashew nuts and mint. Divide the rice between two plates and add the turkey skewers. Serve with lime quarters.

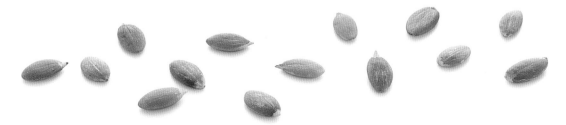

OSTEOARTHRITIS

Reduce red meat and eat plenty of pure foods rich in bone-strengthening calcium.

What is osteoarthritis?

A wear-and-tear arthritis, osteoarthritis causes the cartilage that lines your joints to break down, creating inflamed joints and stiffness. Changes in the cartilage trigger the growth of more bone, leading to joint deformities and more pain.

Pure-food solutions

EAT FEWER DEADLY NIGHTSHADES Deadly nightshades – including tomatoes, aubergine (eggplant), (bell) pepper, chilli, white potato and tobacco – can irritate joints and inflammation. Try removing them from your diet.

REDUCE CAFFEINE Caffeine disturbs calcium metabolism and can lead to a drastic calcium reduction in your bones. Avoid it; or at worst drink decaff. Sulphur-rich foods (onions, garlic, asparagus) help the body to absorb calcium.

EAT MORE PINEAPPLE Fresh pineapple (not tinned) contains a protein-digesting enzyme called bromelain, which can help to reduce inflammation and pain in swollen joints. Add it to your fruit salads regularly.

EAT MORE ALKALINE FOODS The more alkaline your blood, the less likely you are to experience pain. Watermelon, lemons, dates, figs, seedless grapes and watercress are among good alkalizing foods. Red meat, sugar and white-flour products (the usual suspects!) are among the most acidic – avoid them.

EAT PLENTY OF CALCIUM-RICH FOODS Foods rich in calcium will help to prevent your bones becoming brittle, so try to maximize them in your diet. The top calcium-rich foods include mackerel and salmon with bones, green leafy vegetables, dried figs, tofu, broccoli, beans, sesame seeds (unhulled tahini), quinoa and almonds.

MAXIMIZE YOUR INTAKE OF OMEGA-3 FOODS Foods rich in omega-3 essential fatty acids help to reduce inflammation and pain in your joints. To increase your intake of omega-3, the best foods to eat include cold-pressed, organic canola, fish, hemp, soybean and linseed (flax seed) oils; dark leafy green vegetables; pumpkin seeds; walnuts; mackerel; herring; and salmon.

Spinach salad with spiced sweet potato croutons

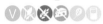

SERVES 2
PREPARATION TIME 20 MINUTES
COOKING TIME 20 MINUTES

1 large sweet potato (350g/12oz), peeled and cut into 1cm/½in cubes
1 tbsp extra virgin olive oil
¼ tsp ground cumin

110g/4oz tofu
3 tbsp water
4 tsp lime juice
1 tsp fresh ginger, grated
2 large handfuls (120g/4oz) baby spinach leaves
6 salad onions, trimmed and finely sliced
1 tbsp unsalted pistachio nuts, halved and lightly toasted

1 Preheat the oven: 200°C/fan 180°C/400°F/gas 6.

2 Put the potato, olive oil and cumin in a large bowl and toss to coat the potato thoroughly. Transfer to a large baking sheet and spread out. Roast in the top of the oven for 20 minutes, turning the cubes over halfway through.

3 Meanwhile put the tofu, water, lime juice and ginger in a blender. Blitz until smooth. Add a little extra water if the dressing is too thick – it should be the consistency of single cream.

4 Put the spinach and onions in a bowl. Pour over the tofu dressing and toss. Scatter over the pistachio nuts and the potato croutons to serve.

NOTE: Silken tofu is ideal for this dressing. It can be wetter than ordinary tofu so use 1 tbsp water and add more water if necessary.

PRE-MENSTRUAL SYNDROME (PMS)

Boost your intake of zinc and chromium and reduce the toxins in your diet.

What is PMS?

In a normal menstrual cycle, levels of the hormones estrogen and progesterone rise and fall in a balanced, healthy way. When there is an imbalance, PMS results. In addition, fluctuating blood sugars, stress and poor liver function can all exacerbate the symptoms (see supplements, opposite) of PMS.

Pure-food solutions

INCREASE THE MINERALS Found in foods such as organic eggs and chicken, zinc keeps the reproductive system healthy and is a vital component of insulin, which regulates blood sugars. Chromium, found in brown rice and chicken, and magnesium (see p.181) also help to regulate sugar levels. Magnesium also relaxes the muscles, so can ease cramping.

EAT LIVER-FRIENDLY FOODS The liver breaks down estrogen, which is critical in PMS associated with high estrogen levels (see supplements, opposite). However, the strain of modern diets on the liver (see p.81) tires it out so that it does not do a good job of breaking down the estrogen. Reduce the load on your liver by eating a chemical-free, pure-foods diet.

Supplements to balance hormones

- If your PMS is triggered by high estrogen levels (symptoms include painful or heavy periods, fluid retention, anxiety and mood swings), try agnus castus. This herb stimulates the production of leutenizing hormone, which in turn triggers progesterone production, balancing out the body's levels of estrogen.
- If your PMS is triggered by low estrogen levels (symptoms include an irregular or extended cycle, depression and constipation), try black cohosh. This herb contains phytoestrogens, plant chemicals that mimic the action of the hormone estrogen. These trick the body into believing that it has adequate estrogen to balance out the progesterone.

Nabeyaki udon pot

SERVES 2
PREPARATION TIME 15 MINUTES
COOKING TIME 40 MINUTES

1 sheet kombu (a Japanese edible seaweed)
1 small shallot (scallion), peeled and thinly sliced
1 small knob (15g/½oz) fresh ginger, thinly sliced
1 fat clove garlic, peeled and thinly sliced
750ml/25 fl oz/3⅛ cups water

110g/4oz buckwheat noodles
2 tbsp wheat-free tamari
1 medium carrot, peeled and thinly sliced
1 small onion, peeled and thinly sliced
225g/8oz skinless organic turkey breast, sliced into thin strips
Large handful (55g/2oz) spinach
4 sprigs coriander (cilantro), to serve
2 salad onions, trimmed and finely sliced, to serve

1 Put the kombu, shallot (scallion), ginger, garlic and water into a medium saucepan. Place over a medium heat, bring up to a simmer and cook for 30 minutes. Meanwhile, cook the noodles in boiling water for 2 minutes, then drain and rinse with cold water.

2 Strain the kombu stock – you should have about 450ml/16 fl oz/1¾ cups (if less, top up with water). Return the stock to the saucepan and stir in the tamari. Add the carrot and onion, place over a medium heat and bring up to a simmer. Cover the saucepan and cook for 4 minutes.

3 Add the turkey, re-cover the pan and cook for a further 3 minutes, then add the blanched noodles and spinach and simmer for a final 2 minutes. Ladle the soup into large bowls and serve with the coriander (cilantro) leaves and salad onions sprinkled on top.

STRESS

Eat pure foods rich in the mineral magnesium and in the B-vitamins.

What is stress?

Stress is often seen as an emotional or psychological problem, but it has very real physical effects. The physical and biochemical changes initiated in stress are largely governed by the adrenal glands, which release hormones called corticosteroids. The hormonal release causes a sudden surge in energy that puts us into the "fight-or-flight" response (see p.119). This heightened state of physical and mental alertness uses up valuable nutrients and places a strain on many of the body systems, including digestion and the heart and circulation. In the long term this extra strain takes its toll on the body, causing illnesses that can be as serious as heart disease and cancer.

Pure-food solutions

EAT MORE MAGNESIUM-RICH FOODS Prolonged stress reduces magnesium in the muscles, leading to muscle fatigue, headaches and cramps. Eating magnesium-rich foods (see p.181) can help to replenish the supply.

STOCK UP ON B-VITAMINS Enervation, a naturopathic philosophy, occurs when stress wears down the nervous system, creating a state of exhaustion. Rest and regular exercise will help, but so will pure foods rich in the B-vitamins, which energize the nervous system. These foods include whole grains (rice, amaranth, quinoa, rye, oats and spelt), fresh vegetables (especially yams, onions, garlic and dark green vegetables) and fresh fruit.

Vegetarian buckwheat yakisoba

SERVES 2
PREPARATION TIME 20 MINUTES
COOKING TIME 14 MINUTES

110g/4oz buckwheat soba noodles

2 tbsp extra virgin olive oil

1 clove garlic, peeled and crushed

1 tsp fresh ginger, grated

1 small onion, peeled and thinly sliced

1 medium carrot, peeled and cut into matchsticks

2 handfuls broccoli florets

2 tbsp water

2 handfuls oyster mushrooms (110g/4oz),
halved if large

¼ medium savoy cabbage (110g/4oz), shredded

3 tbsp wheat-free tamari

2 tsp sesame oil

1 Cook the noodles in boiling water for
4–5 minutes, until just tender. Drain and
rinse with cold water.

2 Pour the oil into a wok and place over a high
heat. Add the garlic, ginger, onion, carrot,
broccoli and water and stir-fry for 2 minutes.
Add the mushrooms and cook for 3 minutes,
then add the cabbage and cook for a further
2 minutes, until all the vegetables are tender.

3 Add the noodles and cook for 1–2 minutes to
heat through. Stir in the tamari and sesame oil
just before serving.

MAX'S STRESS-BUSTING TEA

Many herbs have a wonderful, restorative effect on the
nervous system, helping to relieve stress and bring back
lost energy. Try a tea based on equal parts of the herbs
passionflower (*Passiflora*) and licorice (*Glycyrrhiza
glabra*), which will help to give you a sense of calm and
also give your exhausted adrenals a boost. Mix the
dried, organic herbs together and then use one
teaspoon per cup of tea. Allow the tea to steep for five
minutes in boiling water and then sip slowly. If you like,
you can add half a part Siberian ginseng
(*Aleutherococcus senticosus*), too.

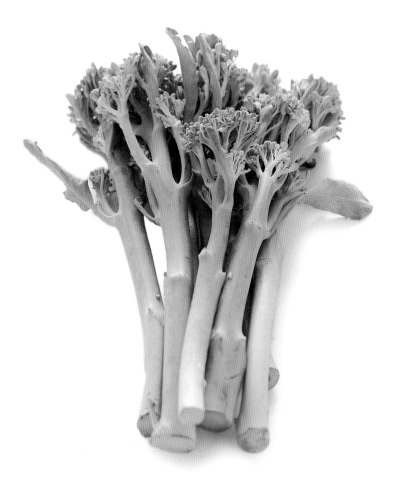

WATER RETENTION

Reduce salt and saturated fat, and eat pure foods rich in bioflavonoids and chlorophyll.

What is water retention (edema)?

Your body is 70 per cent water and has two main fluid transport systems – the blood and the lymph. If either of these systems is not functioning at optimum levels, fluid builds up in the tissues, leading to water retention. Excess water in the body raises blood pressure, puts a big strain on the kidneys and affects the fine balance of minerals in your blood, lymph, cells and tissues. The bloating can also cause muscle aches and pains. Long-term, persistent water retention can indicate a problem with the kidneys, bladder, heart or liver.

Pure-food solutions

EAT GOOD FATS One of the main causes of edema is high blood pressure, which forces fluid out of the veins and arteries and into the surrounding body tissues, where it accumulates. High blood pressure can be the result of hardened fatty deposits, known as plaques, on the insides of the arterial walls. Reducing your intake of saturated animal fats, such as those in butter, cream and bacon, can help to prevent the plaque formation, while an increase in the blood-thinning omega-3 fatty acids, found in foods such as fresh salmon and ground linseeds (flax seeds), helps to lower blood pressure and reduce edema.

INCREASE BIOFLAVONOIDS These compounds help to maintain the health of the veins and arteries, preventing fluid leaking out into the body's tissues. They occur in (bell) peppers, buckwheat, blackcurrants, apricots, citrus fruits and grapes. Try to eat four portions of these foods each week.

CUT OUT SALT Salt creates water retention. High levels of salt (sodium chloride) in the body attract water into the cells, leading to a fluid build-up. To reduce your salt intake (we need fewer than 500mg a day), stop using salt in your cooking and stay away from processed foods. Garlic is a great substitute for salt as it enhances flavour as well as improving lymph and blood circulation.

EAT MORE "GREEN" Chlorophyll, the green pigment in vegetables and fruit, is a potent detoxifier as it stimulates the body to rid itself of excess fluids. A daily shot of wheatgrass juice or big plate of steamed greens will do the job.

Watercress soup

SERVES 2
PREPARATION TIME 10 MINUTES
COOKING TIME 30 MINUTES

1 medium onion, peeled and chopped
3 medium sticks celery, finely sliced
1 medium potato, peeled and cut into small dice

1 tbsp extra virgin olive oil
1 medium clove garlic, peeled and crushed
1 large bunch (85g/3oz) watercress
400ml/14 fl oz/1⅔ cups vegetable stock
25 gratings nutmeg

1 Put the onion, celery, potato and olive oil in a large saucepan. Cover with a lid, place over a low heat and cook very gently for 20 minutes. Stir the mixture occasionally to prevent the vegetables from sticking.

2 Uncover the pan, add the garlic and cook for 1 minute. Reserve a large handful of watercress and add the rest of the bunch to the pan with the stock. Increase the heat to medium, bring up to a simmer and cook for 10 minutes.

3 Transfer the soup to a blender and allow to cool slightly. Add the reserved watercress and whiz until smooth – when blending, take care that the hot liquid does not splash you. Return the soup to the saucepan and season with the nutmeg. Reheat gently before serving.

NOTE: You can serve each bowl of soup with a teaspoon of live goat's yogurt swirled on top if you like. You can also sieve the soup after blending for a very smooth texture, but be aware that you will lose some of the fibre.

15 FURTHER AILMENTS AND THEIR PURE-FOOD SOLUTIONS

This table lists a further 15 common ailments and the nutrients you need, foods you should eat and foods you should avoid when trying to regain your health. If your symptoms worsen, please consult your naturopath or doctor.

AILMENT	NUTRIENTS YOU NEED	FOODS TO EAT	FOODS TO AVOID
Anemia	Vitamins C, E, B-complex (including especially B9/folic acid and B12), iron	apples, apricots, asparagus, bananas, broccoli, egg yolks, leafy greens, parsley, peas, plums, prunes, raisins, squash, whole grains	Almonds, cashews, chocolate, cocoa, rhubarb, kale, spinach, beans, beer, ice cream, cow's dairy, coffee
Attention deficit disorder	Quercetin, calcium, magnesium; vitamins B-complex, C	Most fresh fruits and vegetables, wheat-free wholemeal breads and pasta, brown rice	Artificial colours, flavours and preservatives; carbonated drinks; almonds, apricots, apples, cherries, currants, berries, plums, prunes, tomatoes, cucumber, oranges
Bronchitis	Beta-carotene; vitamins A, C, E; bromelain, zinc	Pineapple, onions, garlic, fresh fruit and vegetables, whole grains, oily fish	Dairy products, sugar, junk foods, white flour, beans, cabbage, cauliflower
Cholesterol	Apple pectin, co-Q10, lecithin; vitamins B1, B3, C; fibre, chromium	Apples, bananas, carrots, cold-water fish, garlic, grapefruit, olive oil, whole grains, brown rice, oats, cold-pressed oils	Saturated animal fats, coconut oil, palm kernel oil, sugar, nuts, alcohol, coffee, tea
Cold sores	L-lysine, zinc; vitamins A, B-complex, C, E	Raw vegetables, live-culture yogurt, fresh cod, sardines, tofu, spirulina, nuts, eggs	Sugar, alcohol, refined white flours, sweets, fizzy drinks, wheat
Constipation	Vitamins B-complex, C; probiotics, apple pectin, magnesium, EFAs	Prunes, figs, raw green leafy vegetables, brown rice, whole oats, asparagus, carrots, peas, apples, citrus fruit	Fried foods, saturated animal fats, cow's dairy, spicy foods

AILMENT	NUTRIENTS YOU NEED	FOODS TO EAT	FOODS TO AVOID
Gout	EFAs; vitamins B-complex, C	Raw fruits and vegetables (except those to avoid), nettle tea, celery juice	Meat, alcohol, fried foods, roasted nuts, sugar, white flour, coffee, cauliflower, lentils, fish, eggs, spinach
Heart disease	Co-Q10, calcium, magnesium, L-carnitine, lecithin, vitamin E, omega-3 fats, selenium, phosphatidyl choline	Whole grains, skinless turkey, skinless chicken, garlic, onions, apples, olive oil, salmon, tuna, trout, mackerel, raw fruits and vegetables	Salt, caffeine, saturated animal fats, white flour, sugar, alcohol, spicy foods
Hypothyroid	L-tyrosine, B-complex, EFAs	Egg yolks, parsley, apricots, dates, prunes, fish, chicken	Sugar, Brussels sprouts, peaches, pears, spinach, turnips, cabbage, broccoli, white flour
Infertility	Selenium, zinc; vitamins C, E; EFAs	Eggs, fish, mushrooms, pecans, Brazil nuts, herring, whole grains, sesame seeds	Alcohol, tobacco, coffee, saturated animal fats, fried foods, sugar
ME and chronic fatigue	Probiotics, co-Q10, magnesium, manganese; vitamins A, B-complex, C, E	Whole grains, brown rice, raw nuts, raw seeds, cold-water fish, live-culture yogurt, kefir, dark green leafy vegetables	Shellfish, fried foods, junk foods, coffee, tea, sugar, sweets, cakes, wheat, cow's dairy
Menopause	EFAs, digestive enzymes with hydrochloric acid, lecithin; vitamins B-complex, E	Broccoli, dandelion greens, kelp, salmon with bones, tofu, tempeh, soya (soy) milk, sage	Dairy products, meat, alcohol, coffee, spicy foods, salt
Osteoporosis	Boron, calcium, glucosamine, magnesium, silica, copper, zinc; vitamin D	Alfalfa, dandelion greens, parsley, broccoli, hazelnuts, sesame seeds (unhulled tahini), whole grains, garlic, onions	Coffee, tea, soft drinks, sugar, almonds, spinach, rhubarb, cashews
Prostatic hypertrophy	Vitamins B-complex, E; zinc, selenium, EFAs	Tomatoes, raw pumpkin seeds, green leafy vegetables, herring, pecans	Saturated animal fats, alcohol, coffee, spicy foods
Urinary tract infection	EFAs; vitamins B-complex, C, E	Seeds, whole grains, raw fruit and steamed vegetables, ground raw nuts, oats, live culture yogurt, ginkgo biloba herbal tea, oat bran	Alcohol, saturated animal fats, salt, sugar, fried foods, burned foods, foods that are cooked in aluminium (aluminum) pots

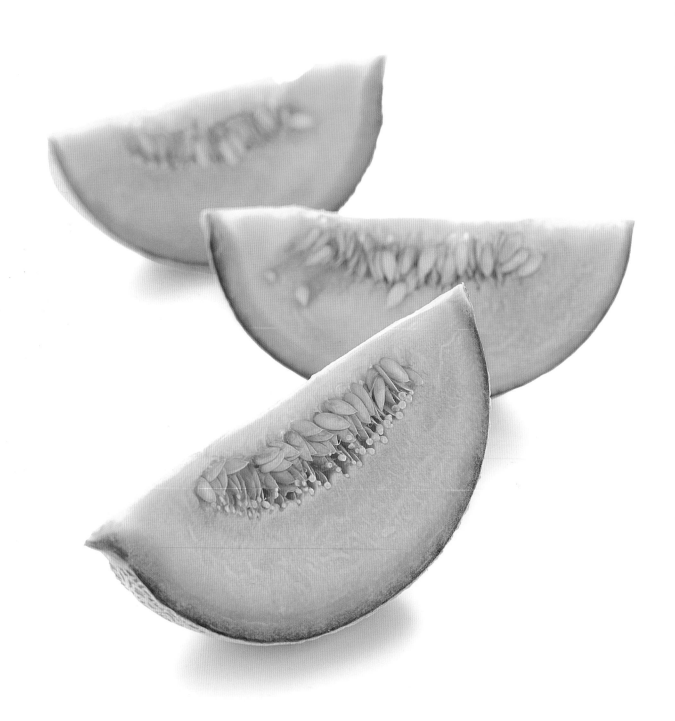

CHAPTER 6

The optimum health plan

If there is one thing that most of us would agree upon, it's that we would love to achieve optimum health – a state of wellbeing that promotes a long life, in which we look, feel and are, quite simply, on top of the world. In this chapter we explore the ways in which you can use a clean diet of pure foods to defy the passing of time – to make you look and feel younger. This includes a specially devised "young-living plan", which lasts a month and optimizes the diet for a younger you. In addition, as good nutrition is only one part of living a pure-foods lifestyle, we look at the five fundamental lifestyle factors that work together with improvements in your diet to bring the best results in terms of health, happiness and looking great – these are exercise, stretching, breathing, relaxing and, last but by no means least, having fun. Enjoy, live long and be happy!

STAYING YOUNG AND HEALTHY

Who says that you can't feel 20 when you're 60? Your body is only
as old as your lifestyle makes it – the years may pass, but we all
have the power to make their passage more cruel or more kind on
our physical and mental wellbeing. Here's how to make them kind.

What age does to us

As we age, our body's internal biochemical processes slow down, the major
organs, including the organs of digestion, begin to wear out, and the body
cannot keep up the rate of cell renewal necessary to keep itself in peak,
youthful condition. A victim and a perpetrator of ageing is the digestive tract,
which over time becomes less efficient at breaking down foods and assimilating
nutrients. The body responds to this reduced nutrient intake by sending any
nutrients it does receive to our vital organs, such as the heart, as a matter of
priority, sacrificing the health of our hair, skin and nails, which we can live
without. The results are the visible signs of ageing – clear warning signals that
you are not getting the nutrients you need to stay young.

As well as the effects on our body, ageing also affects the mind – how many
times have you attributed a lapse of memory to the onset of "old age"?
Mental acuity is based on the availability of nutrients and oxygen in the brain,
with good digestion and healthy blood circulation ensuring a ready supply.

The great news is that we do not have to age as fast biologically or mentally
as we do chronologically. A pure-foods diet slows ageing. It maximizes nutrient
intake so that the body can continue to manufacture new cells, and keeps the
digestion and heart sending nutrients and oxygen to the brain.

Pure-food solutions

LOOK AFTER YOUR DIGESTIVE SYSTEM Many people suffer with the tell-tale symptoms of poor digestion as they get older – indigestion, heartburn, constipation and diarrhea. If your digestive tract is healthy, it will assimilate and absorb the maximum nutritional value from your food, and keep you younger longer. Have a look at the Digestion Tune-up plan in Chapter 3 and take any steps necessary to bring your digestion back to health, or to keep it on the right track well into old age.

LOOK AFTER YOUR NERVOUS SYSTEM A deficiency in vitamin B12 can lead to some of the signs of ageing: weakened limbs, memory loss, mood changes, disturbed balance, lack of co-ordination, and disorientation. A diet rich in lean protein (fresh fish, organic chicken and lean red meat) and tempeh (a fermented soy bean product) ensures a good supply of B12. Good-quality protein is also used to make neurotransmitters, the chemicals that carry the messages through the nervous system, and is essential for mental performance.

LOOK AFTER YOUR BRAIN Low blood-glucose levels can lead to mental confusion. The primary source of glucose (sugar) energy for the brain comes from carbohydrates, so eat plenty of whole grains and fresh fruits and vegetables. In addition, the brain is more than 60 per cent fat. A lack of omega-3 essential fatty acids in your diet can lead to depression, poor memory, and many more mental disorders. To ensure that your diet is rich in omega-3 fats, eat plenty of fresh, organic oily fish such as salmon, sardines, trout, tuna, herring, mackerel and anchovies. In addition, consider taking a supplement of the medicinal herb ginkgo biloba, which stimulates circulation and is especially well-known for its ability to restore blood supply to the brain.

LOOK AFTER YOUR SKIN, HAIR AND NAILS Scientists now believe that many of the visible (and invisible) signs of ageing are a result of free-radical action (see p.36) on the body: the free radicals destroy the body's cells, including those that make up our skin, hair and nails. Pure foods contain natural chemicals called antioxidants, which neutralize free radicals, preventing them from causing damage. Pack your diet with vitamins C and E and the minerals selenium and zinc (see p.198) to maximize your intake of antioxidants.

TEN BASIC RULES FOR A YOUNG YOU

Keeping our body in optimum condition late into our lives does not have to be difficult. If we follow a few simple principles of optimum nutrition, the body will receive all the nutrients it needs to work at its best and, quite simply, we will stay younger longer.

1 Know your food groups

One of the keys to staying young and healthy is to make sure that the body gets a full range of nutrients. To eat a balanced diet might sound like a broad piece of advice, but it also has broad benefits, maintaining the health of all the body systems and the mind. Use the "pyramid" opposite as a guide to eating healthily. Try to cut out the foods at the top of the pyramid, in the red section. Aim for one good-sized portion of each of the amber foods every day, and aim for five portions of fruits and vegetables (the green section) daily.

2 Get your daily dose of antioxidants

Free radicals, or "oxidants" (see p.36), are seen by some scientists as the primary cause of ageing and age-related disease. They are created in the body by the natural biochemical processes of life, by stress and by chemical pollution. Antioxidants destroy free radicals. The main antioxidants are vitamin C (found in high levels in kiwi, oranges, tomatoes, broccoli, cabbage and cauliflower), vitamin E (avocado, eggs, nuts, sunflower seeds, whole grains, green leafy vegetables), selenium (Brazil nuts, sesame seeds, fish, whole grains) and zinc (eggs, herring, mushrooms, turkey, pecans, pumpkin seeds). Green tea contains

THE TRAFFIC-LIGHT PYRAMID OF FOODS

RED: TOXIC – STOP!

SUGAR, SWEETS, JUNK AND FRIED FOODS, SATURATED FAT, CHEESE, SALT, WHITE FLOUR, MARGARINE, ALCOHOL, BURNED FOOD, HYDROGENATED OILS

AMBER: IN MODERATION

WHOLE GRAINS (brown rice, wholemeal pasta and bread), **LIVE YOGURT, PROTEIN** (fresh fish, lean red meat, organic chicken, tofu, beans), **NUTS, SEEDS, COLD-PRESSED OILS, STARCHY VEGETABLES** (potatoes, carrots, parsnips), **GOAT'S AND SHEEP'S DAIRY** (cheese, milk), **EGGS, BEANS, LEGUMES**

GREEN: GO FOR IT!

ALL FRESH FRUITS
GREEN VEGETABLES
(broccoli, runner beans, green beans, kale, cucumber, spinach, cabbage, lettuce, rocket, watercress, pak choi, Belgian endive, Brussels sprouts, radicchio, cauliflower, artichokes, asparagus, mustard greens, and so on)

"Health is wealth. The 'older you' will thank you for looking after the 'younger you'."

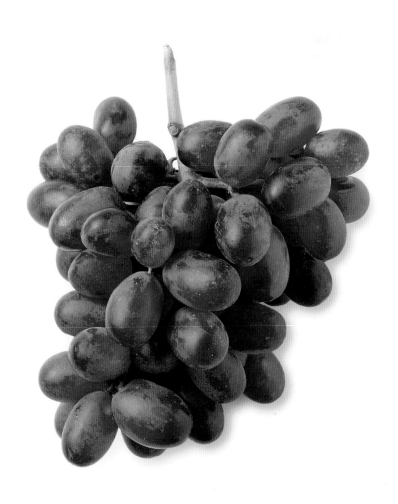

a strong antioxidant called EGCG (epigallocatechin-gallate), and the amino acids in garlic put it at the top of the antioxidant tree.

3 Keep your bowels happy

Modern diets lack the fibre we need to ensure a regular, daily bowel motion. As we already know, if the stool sits in the bowels, we end up toxic and tired. Fibre works by bulking up the stool, making it easier for the muscles in the bowels to push it out. It also sweeps toxins from the intestines, lowers cholesterol levels and regulates blood sugars, helping to prevent heart problems and diabetes. Plant foods and wholegrain pure foods, such as oats, contain the fibre we need to stay fit and young on the inside.

4 Follow the "five-a-day" rule

Aim to eat a minimum of five portions of fruit and vegetables a day. Fruits and vegetables contain not only health-giving vitamins and minerals, including the all-important antioxidants we talked about in Rule 1, but also high proportions of fibre (for the health of your bowels) and complex carbohydrates (which help to keep your brain working properly; see p.197). I suggest having two portions of fruit each day, leaving you to eat three portions of vegetables. Make sure that the fruits are fresh and well washed (especially if they are not organic, to get rid of pesticides on the skin). The vegetables should be raw or lightly cooked (preferably steamed) to ensure that you do not lose the anti-ageing vitamins, minerals and enzymes during the cooking process. As a guide, a portion of fruit is equivalent to one apple, pear, orange or similar-sized fruit; two plums; half a grapefruit or avocado; a handful of grapes or cherries; or a slice of melon or pineapple. A portion of vegetables is equivalent to a medium-sized potato, a large tomato or two medium carrots.

5 Get into phytonutrients

Plant food contains an amazing array of beneficial chemicals called phytonutrients. These healthy, natural chemicals give plants their colour and flavour, and also keep the plant healthy while it is growing in the soil. The humble tomato is known to contain more than 9,000 phytonutrients, many of which have been proven to protect us against disease. The carotenoids in yellow and orange fruits have strong anti-cancer properties, while the purple pigments in grapes protect the heart and lungs. To take advantage of these natural miracles, make sure that your five-a-day (see Rule 4) include differently coloured fruits and vegetables. Time for a rainbow-coloured diet!

6 Go low fat but not "no" fat

Fat has had very bad press over the last few decades and many of us avoid fatty foods altogether. Naturopaths agree that we do not need lots of hard animal fat, such as that found in red meat, cream and butter. We do, however, need some fatty acids, the building blocks of fat, to produce cells, for the transmission of nerve impulses, and in childhood for brain development. A very low-fat diet is as bad for you as a high-fat diet. There are two fatty acids that we need to get from food as the body cannot make them. These "essential" fatty acids (EFAs) are linoleic acid (omega-6) and linolenic acid (omega-3). Sources of linoleic acid include corn oil, nuts, seeds, sesame oil, evening primrose oil, safflower oil, sunflower oil, grapeseed oil and chicken. Sources of linolenic acid include canola oil, linseeds (flax seeds), dark green leafy vegetables, pumpkin seeds, soybeans, walnuts, mackerel, tuna and salmon.

7 Look after your heart

The heart works extremely hard, and to keep young and healthy it needs a plentiful supply of good food and nutrients. Two fantastic healthy-heart foods are garlic and onions. These are known to reduce cholesterol levels effectively and to help prevent blood clots, which can lead to strokes. Omega-3 fatty acids (see Rule 6) also help to regulate cholesterol levels in the blood. Banish salt from your diet as it raises blood pressure, making the heart work harder. Rule 9 has all the facts on salt to persuade you to stop using it for ever.

8 Drink, drink, drink

Only oxygen is more important for life than water. Among other things, this simple, pure fluid helps to regulate temperature, transport nutrients around and waste out of the body, and hydrate the body's cells. The body loses water each day through the urine, the lungs and more than two million sweat glands. To replace it, we need to drink at least 2 litres (4 pints) of water every day, and eat water-rich foods, such as fruit. Municipal water treatment disinfects water, but does not remove most chemicals, so for optimum health it makes sense to filter your drinking water (see p.34).

9 Enter the salt-free zone

When refrigeration was still in the realms of science fiction, we used salt to preserve our food. Nowadays, we use it to "enhance" the flavours of our food. However, we consume far too much salt (most of us need less than 1.5g a day), and anyone who is serious about living a long, healthy life needs to throw away the salt shaker. Table salt, or sodium chloride, is damaging to health because, eaten in excess, it causes the body to hold on to water (causing fluid retention), stiffens the arteries and raises blood pressure. Doctors now agree that we can avoid what was once thought to be age-related high blood pressure simply by making positive changes to our diet and lifestyle. Banishing salt is one such change. Excess salt also places strain on the kidneys, whose job it is to expel unnecessary salt from the body. So, read the labels and avoid foods that have added sodium chloride, or added sodium (multiply the sodium content by 2.5 to get the equivalent content in sodium chloride). Avoid adding extra salt during cooking, and if necessary use lots of fresh herbs and garlic instead to bring out the flavours in your foods.

10 Alkalize yourself

Natural medicine stresses that the body needs to maintain a balance between acid and alkaline to facilitate all of the biochemical reactions we need for life. Modern lifestyles, alcohol, coffee and poor-quality foods push us toward an acidic state. Acidity leads to faster ageing and a marked deterioration in our overall wellbeing. Help is at hand in the form of alkalizing pure foods. A diet rich in fruits, vegetables and water helps to restore the acid–alkaline balance and goes a long way to ensuring longevity and vitality. The best alkalizing foods are asparagus, onions, parsley, broccoli, garlic, okra, squash, green beans, celery, lettuces, sweet potatoes, courgettes (zucchini), lemons, limes, grapefruits, mangoes, papayas, figs, kiwis, apples, pears and all kinds of melon.

THE YOUNG-LIVING PLAN

Are you tired and lacking in energy? Do you look in the mirror and see the tell-tale signs of ageing – limp, dull hair, tiny lines on your skin, hollow eyes? Never fear! I have designed the month-long, young-living plan especially to put the spring back in your step!

What's on the menu?

The young-living menu plan (see pp.207–209) presents a month of pure-foods recipes (some have come from other parts of the book, others have been specially created to be age-busting) that provide all of the nutrients you need to keep your body healthy, young-feeling and even young-looking long into the future. A regular daily dose of plant fibres (from the vegetables) will ensure proper bowel function to eliminate all those harmful toxins, while the powerful antioxidants in the fresh fruits will combat some of the ageing action of free-radicals (see p.36). In addition, a month is long enough to establish some really good eating habits – habits that you will find yourself carrying through into life, well beyond the end of the plan. These habits – such as your daily intake of fruit and veg, steaming your veg, eating healthy desserts, and so on – will set you up for a lifetime of health. I strongly suggest that you add some of the lifestyle advice to your month's eating plan – do a daily regime of breathing, stretching, relaxation and exercise (see pp.214–25) to make sure that your body and your mind stay fit and young.

Daily supplements for young living

The table opposite gives my recommendations for daily supplements to take throughout the plan, or as necessary. You can also use the recommendations as

DAILY SUPPLEMENTS FOR A HEALTHY BODY AND MIND

SUPPLEMENT (DOSAGE)	BENEFITS	CONTRAINDICATIONS/NOTES
Multi-vitamin and mineral (1 tablet a day)	An insurance policy against nutrient deficiencies in your diet.	None known if you take it according to label instructions.
Vitamin C (1000mg twice a day; alternate weekly between the two best forms of vitamin C: ascorbic acid and magnesium ascorbate)	Immune-booster. Needed for the production of anti-stress hormones. Powerful antioxidant. Increases the absorption of iron.	Diarrhea or abdominal pain with very high doses. The body can become reliant on elevated vit-C levels, so reduce slowly if necessary so that the body adjusts to protect you against infection on its own.
Probiotics – lactobacillus acidophilus and bifidus (one capsule containing at least four billion live bacteria, every day before bed)	Inhibit the growth of bad bacteria in the bowels, which can disturb digestion. Also help to manufacture important nutrients, such as B12. Probiotics also promote the proper digestion of food.	None known if you take them according to the label instructions.
EFA oil – a balanced formula containing omega-3 and -6 (1000mg three times a day)	Essential for energy. Promotes healthy skin, hair and nails. Lowers cholesterol and triglyceride levels. Reduces symptoms of PMS.	None if you take it correctly and if the oil is fresh, organic and cold-pressed.
Green formula drink made from plant foods such as sprouted barley, spirulina, chlorella and green algae (1 heaped tbsp in a glass of water or diluted juice twice daily)	Alkalizes the body and supplies natural, food-based nutrients. Rich in fibre and promotes healthy bowel function. A superfood.	None if you take it according to the instructions on the packet.
Fibre supplement (use psyllium husks) (1tsp in a full glass of water per day)	Promotes a regular bowel motion. Helps to cleanse the bowel. Stabilizes blood sugars. Helps to prevent colon cancer.	Ensure that you drink plenty of water with your fibre supplement, otherwise the psyllium will absorb water in your gut, potentially worsening constipation.
Echinacea tincture (When you have a cold: 30 drops in water 3 times daily on an empty stomach. As a preventative: 20 drops in water daily on an empty stomach)	Enhances immune function.	None known if you take it according to the label instructions.
Digestive enzymes (one capsule with each main meal, as needed)	Aid the absorption of nutrients from food. Can calm down digestive bloating and flatulence.	Do not take them long-term as they might mask the symptoms of a digestive problem.

a guide to supplements you can take even when you are not on the young-living plan – that is, as a general supplement regime to ensure that you are maximizing your intake of nutrients every day.

The guidelines I give are by no means a rigid regime, and please do consult a nutritionist or doctor if you think that there may be any reason why some or all of the recommendations could not be suitable for you. If you are pregnant, elderly or suffering from a particular illness, such as heart disease, diabetes or cancer, it is very important that you talk to your health professional before taking supplements. All of the supplements should be available in good health-food stores. As a rule of thumb, try to buy the best brand of supplement that you can afford – like most things in life, you will get what you pay for.

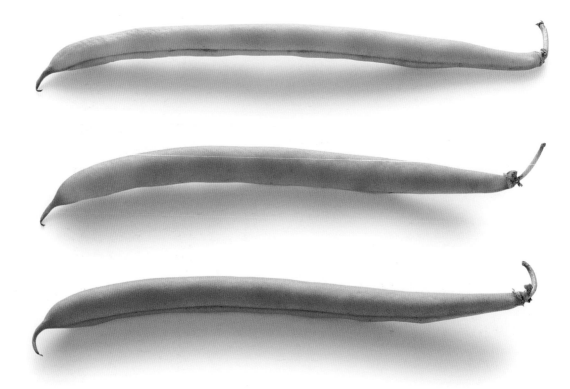

THE YOUNG-LIVING MENU PLAN

DAY 1

Breakfast Aztec porridge (p.140)

Lunch Salmon with fennel, radish and olive salad (p.210)

Dinner Wild mushroom and brown rice risotto (p.150), followed by Papaya and pineapple (p.114) for dessert

DAY 2

Breakfast Scrambled and easy (p.140)

Lunch Winter walnut salad (p.108)

Dinner Stir-fried sesame chicken (p.149), followed by Silken fruit delight (p.153) for dessert

DAY 3

Breakfast Yummy gluten-free crêpes (p.103)

Lunch Warm Puy lentil salad with grilled (broiled) goat's cheese (p.109)

Dinner Slow-cooked pumpkin with canellini beans and gremolata (p.112), followed by Apricot and grape juice (p.104) for dessert

DAY 4

Breakfast Warm linseed (flax seed) porridge (p.102)

Lunch Thai-style chicken soup (p.109)

Dinner Griddled tuna with pineapple salsa salad (p.111), followed by Silken fruit delight (p.153) for dessert

DAY 5

Breakfast The quick cheat (p.141)

Lunch Warm Portobello mushroom, green bean and pumpkin seed salad (p.109)

Dinner Mexican black bean soup with coriander (cilantro) lime tortillas (p.211), followed by Blueberries with lashings of banana sauce (p.152)

DAY 6

Breakfast Warm grain and seed porridge (p.102)

Lunch Refreshing watermelon salad (p.71)

Dinner Mixed vegetable curry (p.151), followed by Papaya and pineapple (p.114) for dessert

DAY 7

Breakfast Proper Swiss muesli (p.141)

Lunch Persian rice with tomato saffron sauce (p.70)

Dinner Bag-baked hoki with spicy tomatoes and steamed green beans (p.150), followed by Mango treat (p.115) for dessert

DAY 8

Breakfast Warm grain and seed porridge (p.102)

Lunch Garlic grilled (broiled) sardines with pomegranate salsa (p.71)

Dinner Warm chicken and blueberry salad with lime dressing (p.149); followed by Macro fruit purée (p.153) for dessert

DAY 9

Breakfast Green fruit salad (p.64)

Lunch Soup au pistou (p.72)

Dinner Teriyaki salmon with glazed vegetables (p.113), followed by Papaya and pineapple (p.114) for dessert

DAY 10

Breakfast Scrambled and easy (p.140)

Lunch Ginger chicken skewers with quinoa tabbouleh (p.72)

Dinner Spring vegetable frittata (p.111), followed by Mixed berries and papaya (p.114) for dessert

DAY 11

Breakfast Warm linseed (flax seed) porridge (p.102)

Lunch Green goddess salad (p.146)

Dinner Griddled tuna with Italian five-bean salad (p.73), followed by Macro fruit purée (p.153) for dessert

DAY 12

Breakfast Yummy gluten-free crêpes (p.103)

Lunch Grilled (broiled) mackerel with Thai salad (p.108)

Dinner Chicken with roast carrots, leeks and fennel (p.113), followed by Papaya and pineapple (p.114) for dessert

DAY 13

Breakfast Warm linseed (flax seed) porridge (p.102)

Lunch Moroccan harira soup (p.146)

Dinner Roast salmon and beetroot (beet) salad (p.74), followed by Mango treat (p.115) for dessert

DAY 14

Breakfast The quick cheat (p.141)

Lunch Steamed salmon with miso (p.148)

Dinner Chicken Waldorf salad (p.73), followed by Creamy rice pudding (p.152) for dessert

DAY 15

Breakfast Warm linseed (flax seed) porridge (p.102)

Lunch Spinach and orange salad with Brazil nut dukka (p.148)

Dinner Really red risotto (p.74), followed by Apple and pear juice (p.105) for dessert

DAY 16

Breakfast Max's muesli (p.65)

Lunch Pure foods pad Thai (p.210)

Dinner Three-bean chilli with avocado salsa (p.75), followed by Pear with red raspberry sauce (p.115) for dessert

DAY 17

Breakfast Warm linseed (flax seed) porridge (p.102)

Lunch Buckwheat crespolini (p.147)

Dinner Stir-fried sesame chicken (p.149); followed by Blueberries with lashings of banana sauce (p.152) for dessert

DAY 18

Breakfast Aztec porridge (p.140)

Lunch Turkey lemongrass skewers with mango rice (p.183)

Dinner Summer vegetable risotto (p.213), followed by Lemon and papaya juice (p.107) for dessert

DAY 19

Breakfast Berry fruit salad (p.64)

Lunch Grilled (broiled) mackerel with Thai salad (p.108)

Dinner Quinoa tart with avocado salad (p.179), followed by Mixed berries and papaya (p.114) for dessert

DAY 20

Breakfast Warm (flax seed) linseed porridge (p.102)

Lunch Warm Portobello mushroom, green bean and pumpkin seed salad (p.109)

Dinner Lemon-baked halibut with garlic-braised chicory (p.173), followed by Silken fruit delight (p.153) for dessert

DAY 21

Breakfast Scrambled and easy (p.140)

Lunch Spinach salad with spiced sweet potato croutons (p.185)

Dinner Griddled tuna with Italian five-bean salad (p.73), followed by Papaya and pineapple (p.114) for dessert

DAY 22

Breakfast Warm linseed (flax seed) porridge (p.102)

Lunch Watercress soup (p.191)

Dinner Teriyaki salmon with glazed vegetables (p.113), followed by Mango treat (p.115) for dessert

DAY 23

Breakfast Yummy gluten-free crêpes (p.103)

Lunch Thai-style chicken soup (p.110)

Dinner Dover sole with shiitake sauce and gingered greens (p.177), followed by Macro fruit purée (p.153) for dessert

DAY 24

Breakfast Warm linseed (flax seed) porridge (p.102)

Lunch Nabeyaki udon pot (p.187)

Dinner Sesame-crusted salmon with stir-fried kale (p.169), followed by Blueberries with lashings of banana sauce (p.152) for dessert

DAY 25

Breakfast Proper Swiss muesli (p.141)

Lunch Warm wild rice salad with griddled tuna (p.165)

Dinner Mexican black bean soup with coriander (cilantro) lime tortillas (p.211), followed by Silken fruit delight (p.153) for dessert

DAY 26

Breakfast Warm grain and seed porridge (p.102)

Lunch Soup au pistou (p.72)

Dinner Tray-baked trout with beetroot (beet) relish (p.163), followed by Pear with red raspberry sauce (p.115) for dessert

DAY 27

Breakfast Green fruit salad (p.64)

Lunch Ginger chicken skewers with quinoa tabbouleh (p.72)

Dinner Pumpkin boulangère with roast chicken and little gem salad (p.176), followed by Lemon and papaya juice (p.107) for dessert

DAY 28

Breakfast The quick cheat (p.141)

Lunch Moroccan harira soup (p.146)

Dinner Grilled (broiled) chicken with nutty millet pilaf (p.167), followed by Mixed berries and papaya (p.114) for dessert

DAY 29

Breakfast Warm linseed (flax seed) porridge (p.102)

Lunch Spinach and lemon falafel with mint dip (p.181)

Dinner Stir-fried sesame chicken (p.149), followed by Papaya and pineapple (p.114) for dessert

DAY 30

Breakfast Scrambled and easy (p.140)

Lunch Rice paper rolls with ginger citrus dipping sauce (p.171)

Dinner Pure foods pad Thai (p.210), followed by Mango treat (p.115) for dessert

DAY 31

Breakfast Aztec porridge (p.140)

Lunch Vegetarian buckwheat yakisoba (p.189)

Dinner Roast salmon and beetroot (beet) salad (p.74), followed by Creamy rice pudding (p.152) for dessert

YOUNG-LIVING RECIPES

Salmon with fennel, radish and olive salad

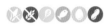

SERVES 2
PREPARATION TIME 25 MINUTES
COOKING TIME 6 MINUTES

1 medium bulb fennel (250g/9oz), finely sliced

2 handfuls (120g/4½oz) radishes, finely sliced

1 small handful (40g/1½oz) Kalamata olives, stones removed and sliced

2 tbsp plus ½ tsp extra virgin olive oil

4 tsp lemon juice

2 x 150g/5oz organic salmon fillets

2 lemon quarters, to serve

1 Put the fennel, radishes and olives in a large bowl. Whisk 2 tbsp of olive oil and the lemon juice together in a small bowl. Pour over the salad and toss well.

2 Preheat a heavy non-stick frying pan (skillet). Brush the salmon with ½ tsp olive oil and cook flesh side down for 3 minutes, then turn and cook skin side down for a further 3 minutes. For better-done salmon, cook for 4–5 minutes each side.

3 Divide the salad between two plates and top with the salmon. Serve with lemon quarters.

NOTE: For extra crisp fennel and radish, soak the slices in a large bowl of iced water for 30 minutes. Drain well and pat dry with kitchen towel before you use them.

Pure foods pad Thai

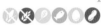

SERVES 2
PREPARATION TIME 20 MINUTES
COOKING TIME 15 MINUTES

125g/4oz medium rice noodles

1 tbsp extra virgin olive oil

170g/6oz tofu, cut into 5mm/¼in cubes

1 large shallot (scallion), peeled and thinly sliced

1 clove garlic, peeled and crushed

1 red chilli, deseeded and thinly sliced (for medium heat)

¼ head Chinese leaf (225g/8oz), shredded

1 tbsp water

3 tbsp wheat-free tamari

2 tbsp cashew nuts, chopped and toasted

4–5 sprigs coriander (cilantro), chopped, to serve

2 lime quarters, to serve

1 Drop the noodles into a pan of boiling water, bring back to the boil. Turn off the heat and stand for 3 minutes. Drain; rinse in cold water.

2 Put half of the olive oil into a wok over a high heat and add the tofu. Stir-fry for 3–4 minutes. Remove the tofu and set aside. Turn down the heat to medium and add the rest of the oil with the shallot (scallion). Cook for 2–3 minutes, then add the garlic and chilli and cook for 1 minute.

3 Add the Chinese leaf and water and cook for 2 minutes. Return the tofu to the wok and add the noodles and tamari. Cook for 2 minutes until the noodles are warm through, then stir in the cashew nuts. Serve with lime quarters on the side, and coriander (cilantro) sprinkled over.

Mexican black bean soup with coriander (cilantro) lime tortillas

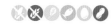

SERVES 2
PREPARATION TIME 10 MINUTES (PLUS OVERNIGHT SOAKING)
COOKING TIME 1 HOUR 15 MINUTES

6 tbsp black beans
1 small onion, peeled and finely chopped
1 tbsp extra virgin olive oil
1 tsp ground cumin

1 clove garlic, peeled and crushed
½ red chilli, deseeded and finely chopped (for mild heat)
700ml/24 fl oz/3 cups vegetable stock
110g/4oz/½ cup masa harina
Small bunch coriander (cilantro), chopped
Finely grated zest of 1 unwaxed lime
110ml/4 fl oz/½ cup warm water
2 tsp live goat's yogurt, to serve
2 salad onions, trimmed and finely sliced, to serve
2 lime quarters, to serve

1   Put the dried beans into a large bowl and cover with plenty of cold water. Leave to soak for 12 hours, or overnight. They should double.

2   Drain the beans and rinse well, then put them in a large saucepan. Cover with fresh cold water. Place over a high heat and bring to the boil. Boil rapidly for 10 minutes.

3   Put the onion and olive oil in a large saucepan and cook over a medium heat for 5 minutes. Add the cumin and cook for a further 5 minutes, then add the garlic and chilli and cook for 1 minute.

4   Drain the beans and rinse them again, then add to the onion mixture. Pour over the vegetable stock and bring up to a simmer. Cover and cook for 1 hour, until the beans have softened.

5   While the soup is cooking, make the tortillas. Put the masa harina in a medium bowl with the coriander (cilantro) and lime zest. Add the warm water and mix to a soft, but not sticky, dough – add more water if necessary. Divide the dough into four balls and roll out between pieces of parchment paper into disks 3mm/⅛in thick.

6   Warm a 20cm/8in frying pan (skillet) over a high heat and slip a raw tortilla into the pan from the parchment paper. Cook for around 1 minute, then flip over and cook the other side for 30 seconds to 1 minute, until starting to brown. Flip again and cook for a further 30 seconds, until starting to brown. Wrap the cooked tortilla in a clean kitchen towel to keep warm, and repeat with the remaining dough disks.

7   Transfer the soup to a blender and allow to cool slightly. Whiz until smooth – take care when blending hot liquids as they may spit. Return the soup to the saucepan and reheat gently before serving.

8   Transfer the warm soup to large bowls and top with the goat's yogurt and salad onions. Serve with the tortillas and lime quarters on the side.

NOTE: Masa harina is special corn flour made for tortillas; don't try to use cornmeal or cornflour/cornstarch. Masa harina is available from some supermarkets and the Cool Chile Co in the UK, and from some supermarkets in the US under the Quaker brand (among others).

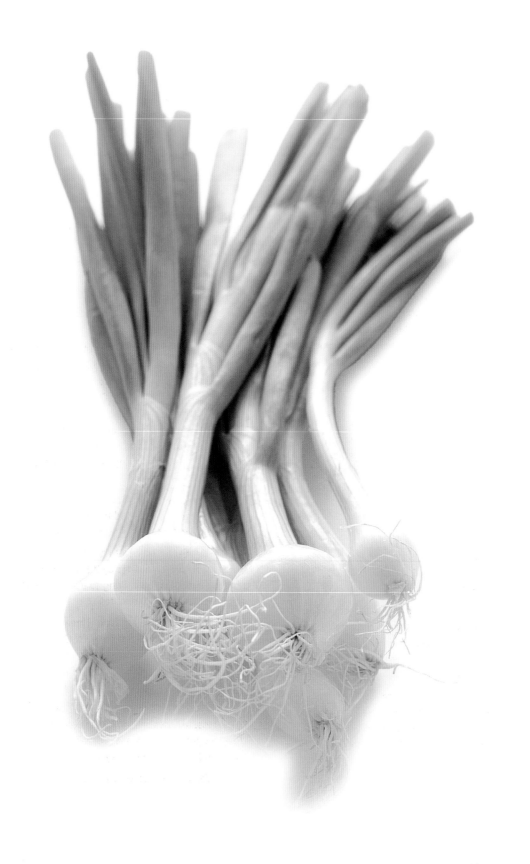

Summer vegetable risotto

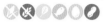

SERVES 2
PREPARATION TIME 20 MINUTES
COOKING TIME 45 MINUTES

1 large shallot (scallion), peeled and chopped
1 small bulb fennel (170g/6oz), halved and thinly sliced
1 tbsp extra virgin olive oil
170g/6oz/⅔ cup brown rice, rinsed
400ml/14 fl oz/1¾ cups vegetable stock
1 medium courgette (zucchini), thinly sliced
Large handful (110g/4oz) green beans sliced into 5mm/¼in lengths
110g/4oz soft goat's cheese, cut into small cubes
5–6 sprigs tarragon, chopped

1   Put the shallot (scallion), fennel and 2 tsp of the olive oil into a large saucepan over a low heat. Cook gently for 5 minutes until the vegetables are just starting to soften. Add the rice and stock, bring up to a simmer, then cover and cook for 35 minutes. Add a little extra stock if the rice becomes too dry.

2   Meanwhile, heat the remaining olive oil in a wok or large frying pan (skillet) and stir-fry the courgette (zucchini) for 4–5 minutes until softened and slightly brown. Set aside.

3   Scatter the sliced beans over the rice, re-cover and cook for 3–5 minutes, until the beans and rice are tender. Remove the saucepan from the heat and stir in the goat's cheese, courgettes (zucchini) and tarragon before serving.

NOTE: Vegetarians can either use a cheese without rennet or 2 tbsp quark instead. This risotto is also a great accompaniment to grilled chicken or fish – just make a half quantity.

Turkey yakitori with sesame millet

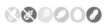

SERVES 2
PREPARATION TIME 20 MINUTES (PLUS SOAKING AND MARINATING TIME)
COOKING TIME 30 MINUTES

110g/4oz/⅔ cup millet
2 tbsp wheat-free tamari
1 clove garlic, peeled and crushed
1½ tsp cider vinegar
225g/4oz organic skinless turkey breast, in 1cm/½in cubes
8 salad onions, trimmed and cut into 1cm/½in lengths
2 tbsp sesame seeds, lightly toasted
2 tbsp sesame oil

1   Soak four wooden skewers in water for 30 minutes. Put the millet in a medium saucepan, cover with boiling water and leave to stand for 10 minutes.

2   Meanwhile, put the tamari, garlic and ½ tsp cider vinegar in a bowl. Add the turkey and onions and toss. Marinate for 20 minutes.

3   Drain the millet and return to the saucepan. Add enough cold water to cover by 2.5cm/1in and put over a medium heat. Bring to a simmer and cook uncovered for 20 minutes.

4   Preheat the grill (broiler) to high. Thread the turkey and onions onto the skewers. Grill (broil) for 5 minutes, then turn and brush with any marinade left in the bowl. Cook for a further 5–7 minutes, until the turkey is cooked through.

5   Drain any excess water from the millet and stir in the sesame seeds and oil and the remaining cider vinegar. Divide the millet between two plates and top with the turkey skewers.

NOTE: You can use brown rice instead of millet.

EXERCISE

Regular exercise is an essential part of the pure-foods lifestyle, helping to promote strong bones, supple joints and powerful muscles. Exercise complements all the good work you are doing with your diet to benefit both your body and mind.

Why should I exercise?

Your body needs exercise, it really does. The old saying "use it or lose it" applies directly to bones and muscles. If you dread the thought of beginning a regular exercise regime, here are some good reasons to change your mind:

- Improved mood and mental performance. Exercise boosts the transport of oxygen and nutrients to the brain, making you feel lighter and happier. It also releases endorphins, the body's natural feel-good chemicals (see below).
- Reduced stress levels. Exercise reduces stress by providing a release for all that excess adrenaline (epinephrine; see p.119). It also triggers the release of the hormone endorphin, which is chemically related to morphine. Exercise can literally work out your frustration and give you a natural "high".
- Increased energy and vitality. Because of the improvements to your circulation, exercise boosts your energy levels. You will feel less tired and lethargic and more ready to participate fully in life.
- Improved sleep. The body is built to move, so if we spend much of our time sitting still, physical tension builds up in our stationary muscles, which then causes restlessness at night. If we work out this tension, we sleep better.
- Weight maintenance, or weight loss. Regular exercise increases our metabolic rate (the rate at which we burn energy), which means that we use up more calories as energy rather than converting them to fat. The result is that at the very least we stop gaining weight, and at most we begin to lose it.

- Improved sugar metabolism and reduced blood-sugar lows. As your metabolic rate improves (see above), you burn up more sugar as energy, steadying the levels of sugar in your blood, giving a more sustained energy release.
- A reduction in unhealthy body fat and an increase in healthy, lean muscle mass. This is the fundamental point of exercise – physical activity burns off the fat and builds up the healthy muscle. Simple.
- Improved flexibility in the spine and joints. When we exercise we move the tendons that join the bones together in all the directions nature intended. The more we move the tendons, the more flexible they become.
- Improved skin quality and texture. We are back to circulation again. Improving blood-flow around the body includes improving it to the skin. This helps to keep the skin supple and young-looking.
- Improved self-esteem. The release of endorphins and the results of exercise – quite simply a better-looking body – will do your self-esteem no end of good.

How should I exercise?

The answer to this has to be "In whatever way you can keep it up!" If exercise is enjoyable, you are more likely to make it part of your regular routine, and stick to it. If you cannot face a sweaty gym, then make sure that you get out and have a walk each day. If you love swimming, but hate the idea of running, throw out the running shoes, find your costume, and swim!

If you have not exercised for a while, start slowly and build up gradually. If you hurt when you exercise, seek medical help. If you suffer from heart problems or any other serious illness, do not embark on an exercise program without first talking to your doctor. Whatever exercise you do, the aim is to raise your heart

WORK OUT YOUR MAXIMUM HEART RATE

When you exercise aim to raise your heart rate to at least 60 per cent of its maximum beats per minute, for around 30 minutes. You can calculate a guideline maximum heart rate by subtracting your age from 220. For example, if you are 40 years old, your maximum heart rate is 220 minus 40, so 180 beats per minute. Sixty per cent of this is 108 beats per minute, which should be the minimum you aim for during exercise.

rate for a short period of time to improve circulation so that nutrients fire their way around your body. Never exercise so hard that your heart exceeds its maximum output for your age (see panel, p.215). The fitter you become, the quicker your heart will return, after exercise, to its normal, resting rate.

There are four main components to a complete exercise program.

WARM-UP Always do a few simple stretches to warm up before exercise. Shake your arms and legs out to loosen muscles. Gently stretch the fronts and backs of your legs and warm up the back and hips by swinging your arms gently to the sides, rotating your back. Flex your neck backward and forward and shake out your arms. Breathe deeply to stretch the abdomen.

CARDIOVASCULAR WORK This type of exercise raises your heart rate and makes you puff and pant. Choose to do something that you enjoy and will stick to – brisk walking, or running, cycling, vigorous swimming, aerobic classes (or an exercise DVD), or a session at the gym on a treadmill. You need to do at least 30 minutes of daily exercise at around 60 per cent of your maximum heart rate to get the benefits of cardiovascular exercise. For most people, this equates to a 30-minute brisk walk, which is definitely 100-per-cent achievable.

STRENGTH WORK Muscle mass and strength decline with age. The only way to maintain healthy, lean muscle is to weight train. Although it is probably easier to do strength training in a well-equipped gym, there are forms of resistance training (a form of weight training) that you can do in your own home. Push-ups, squats, lunges, sit-ups and calf-raises (standing straight, then repeatedly going up onto tip toe and then lowering your heels to the ground) are all easily achievable at home. Try to practise strength training three times a week for about 20 minutes at a time. You may find that your muscles are sore to begin with, but this is just a sign that they are growing. Over time, slowly increase the repetitions or weights, making your workout gradually harder.

STRETCHING AND FLEXIBILITY Weight-training and aerobic exercise can tighten muscles, reducing your flexibility and range of motion. To combat this you must stretch after exercise. Stretching transports oxygen to the muscles, removing the toxins that accumulate during exercise and that cause stiffness. I cover stretching on pages 218–21.

"Do the hard work now – exercise well
and every cell in your body will thank
you by pounding out more energy and
giving you a longer, happier life."

STRETCHING

Regular stretching can help us to defy the passing of time, keeping us flexible well into old age. In addition, regular weight-training can shorten muscle groups, also causing a loss of flexibility. Stretching after exercise will lengthen the muscles again, restore blood-flow, and flex joints. Here's how to stay supple.

Five-minute stretch routine

Taking five minutes out of your day to stretch is a small price to pay for mobility later in life. Over the following pages I've set out an easy stretch routine, which covers all of the major muscle groups and is a fantastic way to wake up your body every morning. It is also the perfect post-exercise stretch, as it helps to cool down the body. Make sure that you are wearing loose-fitting clothing that will not hamper your ability to stretch fully. Breathe slowly throughout – don't hold your breath. We start at the top of the body, and work downward.

Neck and shoulder stretch

1 Stand comfortably. Fix your gaze at eye level ahead of you. Lower your right ear toward your right shoulder Keep your shoulders down. Stretch your left arm down, pushing your fingers toward the floor. Hold the stretch and breathe comfortably. Repeat on your left side. Do this twice on each side.

2 Release your arms and let them hang loosely. Drop your chin to your chest. Feel the stretch in your upper back. Hold for a minute. Repeat twice more.

3 Tilt your head back so that you look slowly up at the ceiling. Feel the stretch in your neck. Hold for a minute, then repeat twice more.

BASIC RULES FOR EFFECTIVE STRETCHING

- Don't rush. Take your time and move gently into each stretch. Hold the stretch for at least 30 seconds.

- Stay relaxed while you stretch. In particular, keep your shoulders relaxed.

- Do not bounce when you are fully stretched, as this can damage your muscles and joints.

- Keep breathing. Holding your breath creates tension in the body and reduces your ability to relax and stretch.

- Relax once you have reached your stretching limit. You may even find that you can stretch a bit further if you relax into the stretch.

- Stop if you feel dizzy or unwell.

Back stretch

Naturopaths say that you are only as young as your spine. A good back stretch brings fresh blood into the spinal muscles, keeping it supple and flexible. This is my favourite back stretch – my cat does it every morning with me.

1 Go down on all fours, keeping your knees and hands shoulder-width apart. Drop your chin to your chest so that you are looking back between your legs. Breathe out and arch your back up gently, pushing the spine toward the ceiling. Hold for as long as you find comfortable without breathing in.
2 As you breathe in drop your stomach toward the floor, curving your spine downward and tilting your head to look up at the ceiling. Hold until you need to breathe out again. Repeat the whole sequence of arching up and down three or four times.

Chest stretch

1 Stand up tall and clasp your hands behind your back. Breathe in deeply and raise your chest while pushing your arms down toward the floor. Hold for a slow count of five.
2 Relax the pose and breathe out. Repeat the stretch twice more.

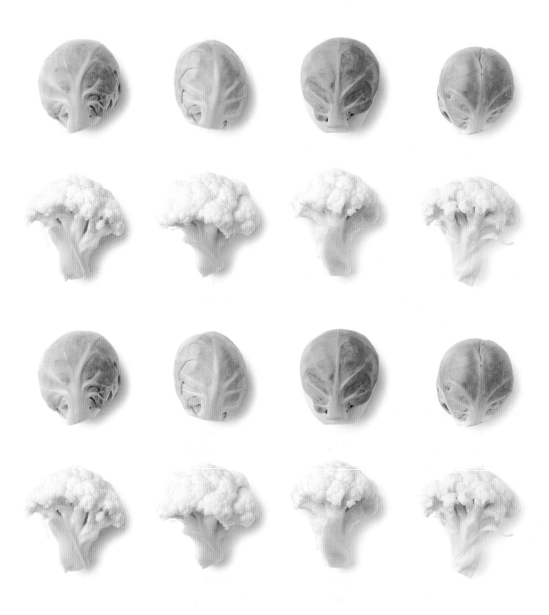

Stretch for the backs of the legs

1 Stand tall, feet slightly apart. Move your left foot forward about a foot's length. Bend your right knee slightly, keeping your left leg straight. Gently suck in your stomach.
2 Lean forward from the hips and place both your hands on your right thigh. Relax your shoulders and keep your back straight. Lift the toes on the left foot up toward the ceiling. Hold and feel the stretch in the back of the leg. Repeat on the other side. Do this twice on each leg.

Stretch for the fronts of the legs

1 Stand up tall, feet shoulder-width apart, shoulders relaxed and stomach pulled in slightly. Bend your right leg and bring the heel up to the buttock. (Hold on to the back of a chair for support if you need to.)
2 Grasp the right foot with your right hand and pull the foot gently into the buttock. Do not lock your left knee, keep it slightly bent. Repeat on the other side. Do this twice on each side.

Full spinal twist

1 Lie flat on your back. Raise your knees, then place your hands on your knees and pull them in toward your chest. Relax your back into the floor.
2 Straighten your left leg. Place the right heel on the left leg, just above the kneecap. Place the left hand on the right kneecap. Stretch the right arm away from the body at shoulder height, palm up.
3 Breathe in and as you exhale use the left hand to gently pull the right knee and leg down onto the floor on your left side. Go only as far as you feel you can. Keep the right foot touching your left knee if you can. Your right shoulder might rise off the ground at first, but as you get more flexible it will stay on the floor. Stay like this for a minute or so, breathing gently.
4 Bring the right leg up. Bend the left leg again and bring both knees in toward your chest. Start the stretch on the other side by straightening out the right leg.

To finish the routine, stand up and shake out your arms, hands and legs.

BREATHING

An old teacher of mine used to say: "Listen to your breathing. Feel it, taste it, savour it and above all enjoy it." Sounds strange until you start to practise breathing with awareness and you realize just how amazing, energizing and liberating proper breathing can be.

Breath – the life force

In naturopathic philosophy, the breath has a more esoteric role than simply providing the body with oxygen. It controls the flow of vitality, or "vital energy", through the body, to give us better control of the mind and emotions. The series of exercises below are designed to improve your awareness of your breath, helping to keep the body and mind in vibrant health. Take a few minutes each morning to practise one of the breathing exercises. When you first begin, you might like to use the Abdominal Breathing exercise to re-teach your body how to breathe properly (you did it naturally when you were a baby!). If you are embarking on a difficult or busy day, use the Calming Breath to focus your mind. If you feel tired and unrefreshed, try not to have a coffee, but rather spend five minutes energizing your body with the Bellows Breath.

Abdominal breathing

If I asked you to take a deep breath, you would no doubt inhale deeply, raising your shoulders and sucking in your stomach. However, this simply squashes the lungs, reducing the flow of air into the body. Watch how a singer or an athlete breathes. They inhale deeply into their abdomens, so that the stomach expands and they draw air down deep into their lungs. This is called abdominal breathing and it is the correct way to breathe. This is how it is done.

1 Lie down on your bed or on the floor. Make sure you won't be disturbed for about ten minutes. Loosen any tight clothing. Place a small book on your stomach, on top of the belly button.

2 Take your mind through the body, relaxing all the muscles. Allow yourself to sink into the floor or bed. Focus on the breath. Feel the warm air entering the nostrils and the cool air leaving.

3 As you breathe in, push the book up toward the ceiling. Imagine that your lungs are expanding right down into the abdomen as they fill with air.

4 As you breath out, suck in your stomach and watch as the book lowers toward your spine. Imagine that your lungs are being squeezed back up into the chest by your abdomen. Repeat steps 3 and 4 for as long as you feel comfortable, staying relaxed and without forcing the breath.

Calming breath

1 Sit comfortably in a chair. Feet flat on the floor, hands resting in your lap, back straight. Take a deep breath. Squeeze in a tiny bit more breath.

2 Exhale slowly through the nostrils and as you do so make a "mmmm" sound in the throat. This creates a slight vibration in the throat, top of the mouth and sinuses. Allow this sound and vibration to relax your muscles, calming your body. The sound disappears as you run out of breath.

3 Contract your ribs and tighten your stomach to fully exhale. Repeat the whole exercise five times, enjoying the sound and vibration.

Bellows breath

1 Sit comfortably. Back straight and feet flat on the floor. Rest your hands on your thighs. Relax your shoulders and straighten your back and arms, pushing lightly down onto your thighs for stability. Close your mouth. Look ahead.

2 Breathe in fully through your nose, right down into the abdomen, then breathe out quickly, pulling in your stomach. Pause for a few seconds. Breathe in again quickly through the nostrils. Repeat 30 times.

3 Tilt your head back to look up. Feel the stretch in your neck. This opens the throat, dragging oxygen deep into the lungs. Repeat steps 1 and 2.

4 Drop your chin to your chest, forcing oxygen into your lungs to stimulate the circulation and send energizing oxygen to the brain. Repeat steps 1 and 2.

RELAXATION

In the UK more than 13 million working days are lost every year as a result of stress-related illness; in the US this figure rises to 550 million working days! Recent scientific research indicated that those who spent ten minutes a day in deep relaxation might live on average three years longer and suffer fewer days of illness than a control group who did not practise any formal relaxation. The need to relax has never been greater.

Relaxation vs participation

I regularly ask my clients, "How do you relax?" The common responses are "Watching TV," "Having a drink/dinner out with friends," "Going to the movies/theatre." However, watching TV, eating out, and visits to the pub or movies are not relaxation. These activities are participation – the active use of energy in the business of living life. Relaxation, on the other hand, is about taking a step back, withdrawing inward for a while and finding a deep sense of peace within. The next step toward your total pure-foods lifestyle is to find something relaxing that you can do every single day. It might be meditation, gardening, oil painting, writing or swimming, but it has to create in you a sense of coming home to yourself, a sense of overwhelming peace, a sense of being apart from the world in a calm space that is just for you.

The benefits of regular relaxation

When the body is deeply relaxed, the heart slows down, breathing quietens and becomes rhythmical, blood pressure normalizes, and blood starts to circulate strongly through the relaxed arteries and veins. Oxygen and nutrients get to the cells properly and waste products are removed efficiently. Our thoughts become more ordered and we have a deeper sense of clarity to tackle the day. The most effective ways to relax are through meditation (see p.131), breathing exercises (pp.222–3), and progressive muscular relaxation (below).

Progressive muscular relaxation (PMR)

PMR involves tensing up a group of muscles as tightly as possible, and holding the tension for a few seconds before relaxing. The real benefit occurs when you then make a conscious effort to relax the muscles: by first tensing your muscles, you should be able then to relax them more than if you just tried to relax them in the first place. Regular, daily practice of PMR really does help you to become aware of the tension in your body – and then to relax it. Ten minutes in the mornings and again before bed will help to calm your mind and body.

Follow steps one to three below to tense and release the muscles in each of the following parts of the body (the parentheses indicate how to tense that part of the body; when you release, just let the tension go): hands (clench your fists), arms (tighten your biceps and lower arms, leaving the hands loose), feet (scrunch your toes), fronts of legs (point your feet), backs of legs (flex your feet), thighs (press your knees into the floor), bottom (clench your buttocks), stomach (hold in your abdomen), lower back (press your lower back into the floor), chest (hold your breath and tighten your chest muscles), shoulders (raise them up to your ears), front of the neck (tilt your head back), back of the neck (press your chin to your chest), mouth and jaw (clench your teeth and lips), eyes, forehead and scalp (raise your eyebrows), and face (screw it up tight).

1 Focus your mind on the relevant muscle group. Inhale and squeeze the muscles as hard as you can. Hold onto the squeeze for the count of 5.
2 Feel the tension. Try to isolate the muscle group and don't tense any other muscles. Release the tension by letting go as you exhale. Feel the muscles relax and enjoy the sensation of the tension flowing away.
3 Stay relaxed for about 10 seconds, and then repeat on the same muscle group one more time. Pay close attention to your breathing, making sure you breathe out as you relax.

HAVING FUN

Life can be so serious. Mortgages, work, kids and the never-ending demands on our time and energy. What happened to spontaneity and laughter? Simple: we are too busy working and thinking to think about laughing. I say, it's time to get the giggle back.

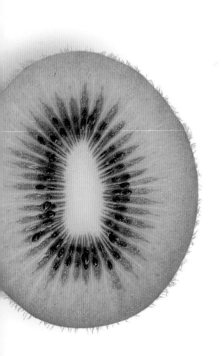

Making time for happiness

Naturopathic philosophy states that all disease has a mental component. The mind and the way we think have a powerful action on our general state of health. A dull, introspective view of life slows down the body, creating an environment that seems to welcome disease and disorder; while a positive outlook seems to attract good health. Having fun could add years to your life, and it is definitely a big part of the pure-foods lifestyle.

However, like everything in life, you have to work to keep happy. You make time to go to the gym to get fit, to visit the hairdresser to get a haircut, and to go to the dentist to check out a toothache. The same applies to fun: you need to set aside time to release your innate sense of joy.

Finding your inner child

One of the best ways to remember how to have fun is to watch children as they play. Children have few or no inhibitions – they don't care if they look silly or get mucky. They live to have pure, uncomplicated fun – splashing in puddles, rolling in fallen leaves, chasing each other, running as fast as they can just to feel the wind on their faces. See how easy it is to have fun? Next time you see a pile of leaves, leap into it. Go on! Jump in feet first – but then let that be just the beginning.

Make a list of what made you deliriously happy as a child. Do it with care, trying to remember and feel the emotions you experienced as a kid. Now make a list of what makes you happy now, or at least what you think makes you happy. Throw away the adult list and go through and do everything on the "younger you" list. Smash through the road-blocks you have set up that stop you from enjoying the pure spirit of being alive.

Do you have a best friend? Everyone needs a best friend. Someone to play with, someone to laugh with. If you have lost contact with your best friend, now is the time to pick up the phone and re-connect. Make time to meet up and have fun. Surprise your best friend by planning a trip away, just the two of you, as mad as your were when you were younger.

When did you last do something that scared you? I don't mean something unsafe or illegal, but rather something that stretched you physically and emotionally. Unlock yourself and step out into adventure. Take your partner go-karting, try rollerblading for a few hours, or go to a rock concert.

Do you have any hobbies? Hobbies are those activities that you do for personal pleasure. Pursue your passions and feel yourself come alive again. Join a group that does something you are interested in. Take an evening course and re-kindle your love of learning. Excite your mind; live your life.

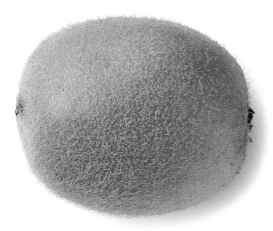 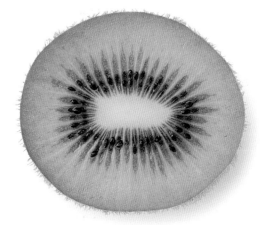

USEFUL ADDRESSES AND WEBSITES

The following organizations will help you to keep up to date and to source the pure foods that make you healthy.

Buying guides

ORGANIC AGRICULTURE

In the UK:
The Soil Association
Bristol House, 40–56 Victoria Street,
Bristol BS1 6BY
T: 0117 314 5000
F: 0117 314 5001
http://www.soilassociation.org

In the US:
Organic Consumers Association
6771 South Silver Hill Drive, Finland,
MN 55603
T: 218 226 4164
F: 218 353 7652
http://www.organicconsumers.org

In Australia:
Biological Farmers of Australia
PO Box 530 - L1/766 Gympie Road,
Chermside, QLD 4032
T: 07 3350 5716
F: 07 3350 5996
http://www.bfa.com.au

SUSTAINABLE FISH

The World Wildlife Fund produce a great guide to buying fish from sustainable sources. You can download it at:
http://assets.panda.org/downloads/fishguideeng.pdf

FARMERS' MARKETS

In the UK:
National Association of Farmers' Markets
PO Box 575, Southampton SO15 7BZ
T: 0845 4588420
http://www.farmersmarkets.net/visit/default.htm

In the US:
You can find a guide to farmers' markets in each state at:
http://www.ams.usda.gov/farmersmarkets/map.htm

In Australia:
Australian Farmers' Markets Association
PO Box 1101, Potts Point, NSW 2011
T: 02 9360 9380
http://www.farmersmarkets.org.au

NUTRITIONAL SUPPLEMENTS

In the UK:
Nutri (Imports & Exports) Ltd
Meridian House, Botany Business Park,
Macclesfield Road, Whaley Bridge, High
Peak SK23 7DQ
T: 01663 718 850
http://www.nutri-online1.co.uk

Nutri-link Ltd
Unit 24, Milber Trading Estate, Newton
Abbot, Devon TQ12 4SG
T: 08704 054002
F: 08904 054003
http://www.nutri-linkltd.co.uk

In the US:
Allergy research group
2300 North Loop Road, Alameda,
CA 94502
T: 800 545 9960
F: 800 688 7426
http://www.allergyresearchgroup.com

In Australia:
Blackmores
23 Roseberry St, Balgowlah, NSW 2093
T: 612 9951 0111
F: 612 9949 1954
http://www.blackmores.com.au

HERBAL MEDICINES AND TINCTURES

In the UK:
Bioforce (UK) Ltd
Brewster Place, Irvine KA11 5DD
T: 01294 277344
F: 01294 277922
http://uk.avogel-server.org

In the US:
Bioforce USA
6 Grandinetti Drive, Ghent, NY 12075
T: 518 828 9111
F: 518 828 9813
http://www.bioforceUSA.com

In Australia:
Bioforce Australia Pty. Ltd.
18 Wadhurst Drive, Boronia, Victoria 3155
T: 006 1398 016755
F: 006 1398 016766
There is presently no website, but you can email bioforce@ozemail.com.au

ESSENTIAL FAT SUPPLEMENTS (OMEGA-3 AND -6 OILS ETC)
Go to:
http://www.udoerasmus.com and follow the links for your country.

RAW FOOD
In the UK:
The Fresh Network
PO Box 71, Ely, Cambs CB6 3ZQ
T: 0870 800 7070
http://www.fresh-network.com

In the US:
Nature's First Law
PO Box 900202, San Diego, CA 92190
T: 800 205 2350 (toll free)
F: 619 596 7997
http://www.rawfood.com

In Australia:
Vitality 4 Life Australia
5/10 Brigantine St, PO Box 1675, Byron Bay, NSW 2481
T: 612 6680 7444
F: 612 6680 7481
http://www.vitality4lifeshop.com.au

Supporting the environment

CLIMATE, SUSTAINABLE FISHING AND CARBON EMISSIONS
The David Suzuki Foundation
Suite 219, 2211 West 4th Avenue, Vancouver, BC, Canada, V6K 4S2
T: 1-800-453-1533 (toll free)
http://www.davidsuzuki.org

REDUCING CARBON EMISSIONS
The CarbonNeutral Company
First Floor, 20 Flaxman Terrace, London WC1H 9AT, United Kingdom
T: +44 (0)8701 99 99 88
http://www.carbonneutral.com

Learning more

NATUROPATHY
In the US:
Bastyr University
14500 Juanita Dr. NE, Kenmore, WA 98028-4966
T: 425 823-1300
http://www.bastyr.edu/

In Australia:
Nature Care College
79 Lithgow St, St Leonards, NSW 2065
T: 02 9438 3333
http://www.naturecare.com.au

NUTRITION
In the UK:
The Institute of Optimum Nutrition
Avalon House, 72, Lower Mortlake Road, Richmond, Surrey TW9 2JY
T: 0870 979 1122
http://www.ion.ac.uk/

In the US:
American Society for Nutrition
9650 Rockville Pike, Suite L-4500, Bethesda, MD 20814
T: 301 634 7050
F: 301 634 7892
http://www.nutrition.org

In Australia:
Contact the Nature Care College
(see contact details in Naturopathy section, above).

Healthy living

IRIDOLOGY, BOWEL AND INTESTINAL CLEANSING
Bernard Jensen International
1914 W. Mission Road, Suite F, Escondido, CA 92029
T: 760 291 1255
http://www.bernardjensen.org

Dr Richard Anderson
About: http://www.cleanse.net
For products:
http://www.ariseandshine.com

HEALTH CENTRES AND RETREATS
Hippocrates Health Institute (Florida, USA)
1443 Palmdale Court, West Palm Beach, FL 33411
T: 561 471 8876
F: 561 471 9464
http://www.hippocratesinst.org

Chiva-Som Health Spa and Retreat (Thailand)
73/4 Petchkasem Rd, Hua-Hin, Thailand, 77110
T: 66 32 511 154
F: 66 32 536 536
http://www.chivasom.com

Contacting Max

If you would like a consultation, or simply want to get in touch to let me know how you are getting on with the plans, I'd love to hear from you. You can find me at:

The Fulham Medical Centre
446 Fulham Road, London SW6 1BG
T: 020 7385 6001
F: 020 7385 3755
Email: Fulham@Max-Tomlinson.com
http://www.max-tomlinson.com
http://www.pure-foods.com

and at:

Welbeck – Pure & Associates Clinic
No.1 Harley Street, London W1G 9QD
T: 020 7307 8735
F: 020 7636 8789
http://www.wellbeckpure.com

INDEX

ACKNOWLEDGMENTS

The Publishers would like to thank Jantje Doughty for design assistance and prop shopping and Sharon Spencer for photography art direction.